"Another fantastic book from Winston and Seif! If you have an active imagination and a nervous system wired for anxiety, you will learn from their eighty collective years of expertise the mindset and strategy for conquering worry and fear. Their book perfectly captures the inner dialogue of the chronic worrier and explains how to retrain the anxious brain to live a life focused on the present; not the past or future."

—**Ken Goodman, LCSW**, Anxiety and Depression
Association of America (ADAA) board member, and
creator of *The Anxiety Solution Series*

"Do you struggle with indecisiveness, catastrophic thinking, or avoidance? Then *Overcoming Anticipatory Anxiety* was written for you. Winston and Seif leverage forty years of expertise empowering all of us into the 'therapeutic attitude,' becoming more observational and metacognitive so we better separate ourselves from our emotional pitfalls. The road map is clear: make cognitive shifts, break the cycle of paralysis through analysis, and you'll no longer fall victim to *anticipatory anxiety*."

—**Josh Spitalnick, PhD, ABPP**, licensed psychologist,
anxiety and obsessive-compulsive disorder (OCD)
specialist board certified in behavioral and cognitive
psychology, and practice owner/CEO of Anxiety
Specialists of Atlanta

"Sally Winston and Martin Seif have written another excellent book—*Overcoming Anticipatory Anxiety*. Traditional efforts to 'cope with anxiety' often mean 'how to get rid of anxiety,' which paradoxically leads to more anxiety. They suggest that allowing and accepting anxiety is a more helpful approach—and I completely agree! I'm thrilled Winston and Seif have written this new book, and I look forward to being able to give it to my patients."

—**Robert W. McLellarn, PhD**, founder and director of
Anxiety and Panic Treatment Center, LLC

"Anxiety can be an uncontrollable, bewildering form of emotional distress that diminishes life satisfaction for millions. Now in this illuminating self-help manual, Winston and Seif unravel the mysteries of anxiety, giving the reader a rare insight into the core processes that drive this unrelenting emotional disturbance. The insights gained from *Overcoming Anticipatory Anxiety* will supercharge the therapeutic strategies of those experiencing or treating anxiety, so they are better able to subdue the debilitating effects of anxiety."

—**David A. Clark, PhD**, professor emeritus at
the University of New Brunswick; and author of
The Anxious Thoughts Workbook, The Negative Thoughts Workbook, and *The Anxious Thoughts Workbook for Teens*

"Sally Winston and Martin Seif have written another compelling and informative book that should be essential reading for those suffering from anticipatory anxiety and chronic indecisiveness. Using evidence-driven principles, the authors provide a unique and clear road map to help people fundamentally change their relationship with anxiety—rather than just managing it—so that they can live fuller, happier, and more meaningful lives."

—**Stacia Casillo, PsyD**, psychologist; and director of
The Ross Center in New York, NY

"Winston and Seif have written another excellent book for people suffering with anxiety and worry! This one offers a terrific explanation of the inner workings of anticipatory anxiety and avoidance, and shows you how to make changes that empower you to live—and thrive—with life's uncertainties. Their description of what anxiety recovery is really like, and answers to common questions, help make it clear how you can change your relationship with anxiety and live the life you want."

—**David Carbonell, PhD**, Chicago, IL-based psychologist
specializing in treating chronic anxiety for over thirty years;
author of *Panic Attacks Workbook* and *The Worry Trick*;
and "coach" at www.anxietycoach.com

"Can you learn to manage your anxiety without practicing hours of exercises? Absolutely! Winston and Seif will persuade you to adopt a simple, powerful mindset that releases you from anxiety's hold. You'll learn as you follow along, and then you'll be rewarded with the life you want and love."

—**Reid Wilson, PhD**, author of *Stopping the Noise in Your Head*

"In their fourth book, Winston and Seif combine their expertise in anxiety treatment to offer insight about the inner workings of the mind. They masterfully identify and describe the phenomenon of anticipatory anxiety which underlies many forms of avoidance and leads to increased anxiety and suffering. What separates Winston and Seif's book is the applicability to not just those suffering from OCD and anxiety, but also to anyone who experiences anticipatory anxiety, difficulty with decision-making, or perfectionism. Their insight may very well provide the key to breaking free from the musings of an anxious mind and offer a guide to leading a more joyful life."

—**Molly B. Schiffer, LCPC**, psychotherapist at The Center for OCD and Anxiety at Sheppard Pratt, and the OCD program at The Retreat

"Winston and Seif have once again contributed a great deal of wisdom to the community of anxiety sufferers. Here, they have teased apart an aspect of the experience that too often gets lumped in with the whole. By singling out 'anticipatory anxiety,' they will surely help the anxious among us understand the role it plays in continuing to feed our worries."

—**Josh Malina**, host of the *Anxiety Book Club* podcast

"Two consummate clinicians, Winston and Seif, put anticipatory anxiety under the microscope in their latest offering, placing it front and center among anxiety phenomena. Anticipatory anxiety is conceptualized as a transdiagnostic feature associated with virtually all anxiety disorders, and therefore warranting a targeted therapeutic focus. The authors offer and deliver a systematic, and well-conceived, approach built upon traditional CBT and Buddhist principles and practices, and guided by biological science. All are integrated seamlessly into an effectively communicated method filled with diverse examples to drive their points home. I will highly recommend this book to individuals who suffer from the potentially crippling effects of anxiety, avoidance, imagined catastrophes, and pervasive indecisiveness—and to fellow therapists alike, who will benefit from the authors' fresh perspectives."

—**Charles S. Mansueto, PhD,** founder and director of the Behavior Therapy Center of Greater Washington, and coauthor of *Overcoming Body-Focused Repetitive Disorders*

"*Overcoming Anticipatory Anxiety* is an informative look at the ways we become trapped in avoidance and anxiety. This instructional guide normalizes experiencing anxiety, reduces shame, and destigmatizes being trapped in this often silent and debilitating struggle. The clear, concise examples and step-by-step solutions on recognizing and working toward freedom from anticipatory anxiety feels like you have Winston and Seif walking alongside and cheering you on as you recover!"

—**Chrissie Hodges, CPFS**, certified peer support specialist; founder of Treatment for OCD Consulting, Peer Recovery Services, and OCD Gamechangers; and author of *Pure OCD*

OVERCOMING ANTICIPATORY ANXIETY

**A CBT Guide
for Moving past
Chronic
Indecisiveness,
Avoidance &
Catastrophic
Thinking**

SALLY M. WINSTON, PsyD
MARTIN N. SEIF, PhD

New Harbinger Publications, Inc.

Publisher's Note

New Harbinger Publications is an employee-owned company

NEW HARBINGER PUBLICATIONS is a registered trademark of New Harbinger Publications, Inc.

Copyright © 2022 by Sally Winston and Martin N. Seif
New Harbinger Publications, Inc.
5674 Shattuck Avenue
Oakland, CA 94609
www.newharbinger.com

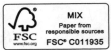

Cover design by Amy Shoup; Acquired by Jess O'Brien;
Edited by Gretel Hakanson

Library of Congress Cataloging-in-Publication Data

Names: Winston, Sally, author. | Seif, Martin N., author.
Title: Overcoming anticipatory anxiety : a CBT guide for moving past chronic indecisiveness, avoidance, and catastrophic thinking / Sally Winston, PsyD, Martin N. Seif, PhD.
Description: Oakland, CA : New Harbinger Publications, 2022. | Includes bibliographical references.
Identifiers: LCCN 2021054431 | ISBN 9781684039227 (trade paperback)
Subjects: LCSH: Anxiety--Treatment. | Cognitive therapy.
Classification: LCC RC531 .W557 2022 | DDC 616.85/2206--dc23/eng/20211228
LC record available at https://lccn.loc.gov/2021054431

Printed in the United States of America

24   23   22

10   9   8   7   6   5   4   3   2   1   First Printing

Contents

Introduction 1

1 Anticipatory Anxiety: Bleeding Before You Are Cut 5

2 Chronic Indecisiveness: Between a Rock and
a Hard Place 31

3 The Biology of Anxious Bodies and Sticky Minds 49

4 Avoidance: How Anticipatory Anxiety and Chronic
Indecisiveness Get Stuck 67

5 Getting Hijacked by Your Imagination 79

6 Fueling Indecisiveness: Perfectionism, Desire for
Certainty, and Fear of Regret 91

7 The Therapeutic Attitude: A Metacognitive Perspective 107

8 Surrender and Commit: The Antidote to Avoidance 127

9 Troubleshooting: Common Questions Answered 149

10 What Recovery Looks Like 159

Acknowledgments 167

References 169

Introduction

Do you often have the experience of dreading an event for days or weeks ahead of time, expecting it will be an ordeal, waffling back and forth on committing yourself to going, planning your potential escape routes or excuses or explanations for failure, making yourself sick with worry? Perhaps it's a social event, or a speech, or a doctor's appointment. Perhaps it's something other people would be looking forward to—your own wedding, meeting up with an old friend, or a chance to travel. Perhaps it's something you have done many times before but just never feel confident about ahead of time—driving somewhere, taking care of your grandchild, or filing your taxes. Do you seek help from others to accompany you or assist you in these situations or to stand by "in case"? Have you become resigned to the repeated and expected experience of feeling anxiety instead of pleasurable excitement before big and small events? Do you get impatient with yourself for being so timid that you miss out on experiences you want? Or are you critical of yourself for having to set up safety nets or for not feeling confident?

If you can identify with these situations, then you suffer from anticipatory anxiety. "Anticipatory anxiety" is the anxiety you experience in anticipation of events or situations that you expect will make you anxious or uncomfortable. Often, it is because they have done so in the past. If you are claustrophobic, when you worry about taking an elevator later in the day, that is anticipatory anxiety. If you have a fear of contamination, when you worry about having to sit on a dirty seat tomorrow, that is anticipatory anxiety. And if you have a fear of public speaking, when you worry that your anxiety will ruin your presentation next week, that is yet another example of anticipatory anxiety.

You may not have heard the term "anticipatory anxiety," but if you experience it, it likely affects your life every day. From your very subtle aversions or avoidances to your most horrendous terrors, anticipatory anxiety is the engine that drives it all. You may have seen its effect on your life and your loved ones. Anticipatory anxiety is what makes you miss out on opportunities, frustrate others with your reluctance to make commitments, and suffer disappointments when you turn down challenges. Anticipatory anxiety is present when you worry, when you back away, and when you try to find escape routes and backup plans. While it's not a formal diagnosis on its own, it is present in almost all anxiety states. Its impact can be enormous, reducing flexibility and diminishing freedom, spontaneity, and pleasure.

But that is not all. Anticipatory anxiety is often accompanied by another set of problems we call chronic indecisiveness—the often-paralyzing inability to make decisions, both small and large. Is there something you have been meaning to buy for years, but every time you think of it, you launch into research that results in no choice made; you find a thousand reasons why you both should and shouldn't buy it; or the whole ordeal becomes too overwhelming or complicated, so you put off the decision once again? Are you at a stuck point in your life—a relationship decision or a job, career, school choice? Have you been wanting to move to another house or city for years and just can't do it? Are you so afraid of either "missing out" or regretting your choice that you cannot decide on any course of action that closes any doors? Do you write pros and cons lists and then do nothing? Do you "know" what you want to do and just don't do it? Or are you afraid of change, commitment, or the unknown to such a degree that you do not progress in your life?

If these conditions describe you, then the insights and suggestions in this book, which are based on contemporary evidence-driven psychological principles, can help free you to live a fuller, more flexible, and enjoyable life. Overcoming anticipatory anxiety can take considerable effort—but it is effort that is well placed. It involves first recognizing when it is leading you to delay or avoid situations and experiences, and then understanding the ways in which your memories, imagination, and desires for safety, security, and certainty can steer you to misleading conclusions about the future. You will learn to identify the role that thoughts and feelings can play in leading you to avoid what you fear, to become paralyzed in making decisions, and to have difficulty differentiating realistic expectations from false alarms. You will learn to treat the signs of anticipatory anxiety as a call to action rather than a red flag signaling danger. And, most importantly, you will learn how to face your fears, make decisions big and small, and live a vital, engaged life.

Why This Book Is Different

You may have read other self-help books and tried various techniques and exercises for relaxation, for getting rid of worries, for making confident decisions, or for how to replace irrational thoughts with rational ones and face your fears. This is not another workbook of techniques. It is not about skill building or *how to*. It is a road map for achieving a fundamental change in your relationship with your mind. It will help you avoid getting bullied by your anxiety and start enjoying the experiences you want. We give you all the information you need to take the leap of faith to move past anticipatory anxiety, to do what you value, and to make choices, large and small, more freely.

It will take effort to identify and understand the ways your brain and body react when you get hijacked by your imagination and feel compelled to avoid. And it will take some courage to try out new ways of doing things. After all, your old ways haven't been successful, and if you want a different result, you will need to try out a different approach. You have likely already put in a lot of effort trying to stop anticipatory anxiety and force yourself to move ahead. We will show you why the kind of effort you have tried does not work well and what works far better. If you follow our suggestions, it will probably be much easier than you anticipate!

We are both specialists in the treatment of anxiety. For the past forty years, we have helped thousands of people learn to overcome crippling anxiety. Our goal is to help you develop an attitude shift, not a set of new techniques to add to the many you have likely tried. This shift is a way to limit the ability of your imagination to convince you that bad things will happen, so you no longer need to limit your life. It is about understanding what is happening so the way forward just presents itself. It is about releasing control and taking your own anxious mind less seriously. It describes a surrender that leads to liberation.

How to Get the Most Out of This Book

This book is intended to be read in the order it was written, from introduction to conclusion. We know that when you are struggling with anxiety, there is always the temptation to turn right to the "what to do" chapters and skip over the rest. But we urge you not to do that. The latter chapters will not make sense without the initial ones, as the underlying processes we describe in the earlier sections give the rationale for how we approach recovery. They also explain why trying harder to face your fears and using willpower to force decisions simply do not work.

Chapters 1 and 2 introduce the concepts of anticipatory anxiety and chronic indecisiveness. In chapter 3, we present the biological underpinnings of anxiety and how they interact with some environmental stressors. Chapter 4 tackles the topic of avoidance—subtle and obvious, big and small, conscious and unconscious—and why avoidance maintains and reinforces anticipatory anxiety and chronic indecisiveness. Chapter 5 explains how your imagination manages to hijack your own good common sense so your predictions become catastrophic and both choice and commitment become problematic. Chapter 6 examines the three major factors that contribute to chronic indecisiveness: perfectionism, the desire for certainty, and fear of regret. Chapter 7 explains the metacognitive perspective that will set you up to move past your fearful imagination and catastrophic thinking. We introduce and illustrate a fundamental shift in attitude that is central to recovery. In chapter 8, you will learn how to apply the shifts in perspective and attitude to real-life situations and be introduced to DANCE—the five steps of therapeutic surrender. Chapter 9 answers common problematic questions that arise, and chapter 10 describes what recovery looks like and how it is maintained.

CHAPTER 1

Anticipatory Anxiety: Bleeding Before You Are Cut

Anxiety comes in many shapes and forms, most of which include anticipatory anxiety as a component. You may have phobias or social anxiety, or you might suffer from panic attacks. Many people have obsessive fears or unwanted intrusive thoughts that cause great suffering. Sometimes anxiety comes in the form of physical symptoms. And, anxiety can just be an ongoing parade of worries that holds on tenaciously and never lets you fully relax. Anxiety is usually accompanied by apprehension about the future and doubts about one's performance, safety, or well-being, and it may affect the choices you make in life. And of course, anxiety constricts your freedom to lead the life you want.

If you have any of these forms of anxiety, then you also experience anticipatory anxiety. In simplest terms, anticipatory anxiety is the expectation of distress and the push toward avoidance that occurs *before* you encounter the situations or experiences you fear in real life.

What Is Anticipatory Anxiety?

Anticipatory anxiety is worry about the future and the fear that bad things might happen or that you might become unable to successfully accomplish what you set out to do. It is the anxiety we feel when we are anticipating a difficult decision, action, or situation. It is how we feel when we buy into our own creative worrying about what bad things could happen. Anticipatory anxiety seems to predict danger; it feels like a warning not to proceed or, at the very least, a warning to proceed carefully.

We think of anticipatory anxiety as a third layer of fear. Let us explain:

1. First, we can be afraid of something. Think, for example: *I am scared of a bee.*

2. Second, we can be afraid of being afraid. This is sometimes called the "fear of fear," and we know this as panic. Think of this example: *If I see a bee, I might get so frightened that I have a panic attack and then lose control or have a heart attack.*

3. Finally, we get to the third level of fear. That is, we can be afraid of being afraid of being afraid. This is not as complicated as it sounds; it goes like this: *I am miserable even thinking about camping next week because I might see a bee and have a panic attack, lose control, and do something crazy. Maybe I should cancel the camping trip.*

You can also think of this third layer of fear as the "avoidance layer." Anticipatory anxiety is a powerful motivator of avoidance because it specifically focuses your attention on the negative things that could possibly happen. If your prediction is only mildly negative—for instance, that you'll sweat a lot when you're presenting your plan in a meeting—then you might believe that you can push through it. But catastrophic predictions—like having a panic attack, making a complete fool of yourself, or damaging a relationship—can lead to incapacitating anxiety that stops you from proceeding. Anticipatory anxiety can make it seem like avoidance is your only choice.

> HELPFUL FACT—Anticipatory anxiety is the third layer of fear and the main driver of avoidance.

Importantly, anticipatory anxiety can also involve expectations not only of anxiety or panic but also of disgust, anger, shame, regret, humiliation, becoming overwhelmed, or any other unwanted emotion. The urge to avoid emerges from the expectation of unwanted feelings from some dreaded failure, loss, or disaster.

HELPFUL FACT—Anticipatory anxiety can involve expectations of any unwanted feeling or experience.

Identifying the Anticipatory Anxiety Component of Your Anxious Distress

Most people have initial difficulty recognizing that the anxious experience has two separate components: there is the anxiety disorder itself (phobia, social anxiety, panic, worry, obsession, and compulsion) and, separately, the anticipatory anxiety. Anticipatory anxiety occurs during the period *before* you expect to encounter what you are worried about. If you are worried that you might have a panic attack in a situation you expect to enter, anticipatory anxiety may start hours, days, or even weeks before the scheduled event. If you are trying to decide if it is safe to meet a new person, or use a public bathroom, or ignore a brief sensation or thought, anticipatory anxiety is the dread you feel when you "try on" that activity or decision and scare yourself with imagining the ways things could go badly.

So how can you differentiate anticipatory anxiety from the dreaded situation, decision, or confrontation it precedes? Keep in mind that anticipatory anxiety varies widely in the way it appears and looks different in different settings. It can present as phobic avoidance, fear of being alone, performance anxiety, or insomnia. It can look like the elaborate planning that someone with obsessive-compulsive disorder must do to avoid encountering contamination or the agony that a person with illness anxiety goes through waiting for test results. It can be the haunting fear of the return of an unwanted intrusive thought. It can also be experienced as chronic hyperventilation. Anticipatory anxiety drives the compulsions that define obsessive-compulsive disorder and related conditions. It is anticipatory anxiety (*I won't be able to stand it if...*) that pushes people to perform the mental rituals and behavioral compulsions to reduce the immediate discomfort caused by the obsession.

Your anticipatory anxiety might be expressed as a fear of going to parties or restaurants or of traveling, lest you encounter something there you believe you can't handle. A desire to avoid being alone at night might stem from anticipatory anxiety about suddenly becoming ill or having scary thoughts. Anticipatory anxiety about imagined relationships might be why you avoid dating. Anticipatory anxiety about possibly getting fired might make you "sick" every morning before you leave for work.

Sometimes people inaccurately label anticipatory anxiety as "free-floating" anxiety. During anticipatory anxiety, your body may be habitually tense, waiting for the event. This can sometimes happen without you being specifically aware of what it is you are anticipating. It can be disabling since having a tense body may lead to headache, chest pain, and muscle spasms. In fact, it is anticipatory anxiety that is the primary driver of chronic hyperventilation (Fried and Grimaldi 1993; Tavel 2017), which is a setup for panic attacks. If you have chronic gastrointestinal problems, such as diarrhea, nausea, or vomiting, they might be directly traced to the anticipatory anxiety you feel (Singh et al. 2016). Anticipatory anxiety may also shape behavior (such as decisions about how to behave, what to say, where to go) in hopes of avoiding a return of symptoms. At lower levels, this fear is like ordinary worry; at higher levels, it may become so intense that it can be called "anticipatory panic."

Anticipatory anxiety is a huge component of the anxiety disorder called GAD (generalized anxiety disorder), a tendency toward unproductive and excessive worrying. What we understand now about GAD is that worry itself really has two parts: an initial worry thought (usually in the form of, *What if [something bad happens]?*) followed by another thought that attempts to make the anxiety brought up by the initial thought go away. This second component gives the illusion of being helpful but is actually the fuel that maintains the anxiety cycle. This is often called "planning," "analyzing," "ruminating," or "coping" by strategizing some form of avoidance. Our earlier book *Needing to Know for Sure* describes this phenomenon in detail (Seif and Winston 2019). Simply put, the imaginative and distressing what-if of GAD is anticipatory anxiety.

HELPFUL FACT—The what-if part of the worry thought in generalized anxiety disorder (GAD) is anticipatory anxiety.

Note: Anticipatory anxiety may be a covert feature of both social anxiety and substance-use disorders, which are often dealt with by taking a drink or a hit *before* leaving for the party or the bar to "get in the mood." Because substance-use disorders and social anxiety often occur together, it is important to tease out anticipatory anxiety as a prominent feature maintaining both problems. Fearful anticipation of distress during withdrawal can maintain addiction. Anticipatory anxiety is also present to some degree in many who do not meet the formal medical criteria for any of these problems.

Anticipatory anxiety is a product of the imagination. It feels like it is a harbinger of what is in store for you in the future, but that is just one of the many ways it tricks and fools you. Even though it is so often completely wrong in its predictions, it is remarkably resistant to change. Understanding this simple truth is the first step to freeing yourself from anticipatory anxiety.

As you read this book from the beginning to the end, you will learn to accurately identify the component of your anxiety that is anticipatory. Many of our patients have told us the recognition that anxiety has two separate components—anticipatory anxiety plus their central fear—has been transformative.

Here is what anticipatory anxiety looked like in one of our former patients with a phobia of flying:

> Molly was a fearful flier whose anticipatory anxiety forced her to stop
> flying for eight years. As she worked to overcome her fears, she took the
> brave step of taking a flight. Then another. Then another. Three years
> later, with dozens of flights under her belt, she has become a rather
> comfortable flier when she is on the plane. However, prior to each
> flight, she still worries about the weather, the health of the pilot, and
> the degree of turbulence she might experience. She also revisits the
> ultimate fear that she might become so anxious that she would give up
> flying altogether.

The point here is that anticipatory anxiety often outlasts the phobia itself. After working on this problem, Molly learned to recognize that the anticipatory anxiety was a false predictor and to not allow herself to consider avoidance as a response to it. She was able to firmly commit to each flight no matter how she felt. Eventually, Molly's anticipatory anxiety subsided when she no longer considered it relevant information to any decisions she was making and treated it like a leftover echo not worth attending to.

> HELPFUL FACT—Anticipatory anxiety is often the last to go during the process of recovery from anxiety disorders and OCD.

While you may not be a fearful flier, the important point is that the anxious anticipation of something feared is often much more debilitating than the situation or experience itself. And, as you'll see below, this experience is extremely common.

How Common Is Anticipatory Anxiety?

There are many studies—population surveys called "epidemiological" studies—that estimate how many people have specific psychological disorders. However, as we noted earlier, anticipatory anxiety is not a single diagnosis. Instead, it is a "transdiagnostic" phenomenon, a pervasive feature of almost all anxiety disorders that is present in many people with mood disorders, especially depression; it is also a feature of post-traumatic stress disorder, particularly in anticipation of confronting reminders of the traumatic event. For that reason, we can't pinpoint how many people are affected by anticipatory anxiety.

So instead, let's look at the numbers broadly. Most studies suggest that—over their lifetime—about 10 percent of the population will develop an anxiety disorder. About the same number will develop depression in their lifetime, and 5 to 7 percent experience post-traumatic stress disorder. If we are extremely conservative, our guesstimate is that 15 percent of individuals will be affected by anticipatory anxiety during their lifetime (Eaton et al. 1981). That is over fifty million people just in the United States.

So, if you are struggling with anticipatory anxiety, you can be sure that you are not alone. Anticipatory anxiety is a pervasive phenomenon, and there is no age group that is shielded from it.

Across the Life Span

Anticipatory anxiety often runs in families. As you read this book, you may begin to notice anticipatory anxiety in your children and older family members. It can appear a little different at different ages.

Once a child is old enough to imagine future events, anticipatory anxiety can flourish. It is the culprit when your child spends weeks dreading getting her vaccination. She may ask a lot of questions about what it will feel like or just be oppositional, crabby, or unable to sleep. The day of the vaccination, when she is in the doctor's office, she may fight, cry, and struggle. The deed is over so fast that everyone wants to say, "See? All that fuss for nothing." But she seems no better the next time. That is because the anticipatory anxiety is often the worst part of the whole experience, and your child remembers the anticipatory anxiety far more vividly than the actual event.

Here are other examples: Your son might beg to not go to his friend's birthday party. But he eventually gives in and—after an initial period of hesitation and shyness—ends up enjoying himself. Or, in the days and hours leading up to their SAT, a teenager may be a bundle of nerves, acting as if nothing is right, rolling their eyes, or picking fights. Or there may be vomiting or a stomachache the night before a concert or before a visit to a noncustodial parent. Or they may not have an appetite for dinner as soon as someone mentions leaving for camp. Typical targets for children include worrying about the health, safety, or death of a parent; starting any new activity; school or camp expectations; and going to sleep alone. For teens, school and peer social issues are prominent targets of anticipatory anxiety as are their worries about their future choices, like college, work, and dating, and even the future of the earth itself.

At the other end of the spectrum, as we age, we become increasingly aware of physical vulnerabilities, unreliable memory, out-of-date technological know-how, and frequently, losses and other unwelcome changes.

Older adults often become more vigilant and have increased anticipatory anxiety. Just one fall or episode of forgetting something important can provoke serious anticipatory anxiety. Many seniors who are quite capable of independent activity and new learning can nevertheless lose confidence and can be dissuaded from engaging in new activities because of their anticipatory anxiety. Typical targets for seniors include walking, being alone (especially at night), health and financial issues, dealing with new technology, reactivity to media events, and fears of disability or dementia.

Anticipatory anxiety acts the same way at any age and with any issue: urging avoidance, making us hesitant, and ruining pleasure. And, as we will show you, the way out of its grip is guided by the same principles regardless of your age. But first let's look at how indecision perpetuates anticipatory anxiety.

The Role of Indecision in Exacerbating Anticipatory Anxiety

If you look closely, you will see that your anticipatory anxiety increases with indecision and decreases with each decision you make. Interestingly, this is true whether your decision is to avoid or, conversely, if your decision is to firmly commit to action no matter what.

Suppose that you are scheduled to speak at a team meeting tomorrow and you are terrified that you will mess up. If you make the decision to call in sick and ask someone else to do that job, then your anticipatory anxiety will plummet. You will feel much more relaxed. You might feel annoyed at yourself—even thinking of yourself as a failure or incompetent—but your terror about the following day will go away. When you decide not to put yourself through the imagined ordeal, the relief floods in. As soon as anticipatory anxiety forces you to avoid, it is gone.

> HELPFUL FACT—Anticipatory anxiety disappears, but sometimes only temporarily, as soon as you make the decision to avoid.

On the other hand, if you keep oscillating back and forth about going to the meeting, constantly debating and changing your mind, you will find that your anticipatory anxiety increases. And, as it becomes more and more urgent to decide, it also becomes less and less easy to do so. There is no relief.

A less obvious phenomenon happens when you decide to commit to the activity no matter what and you do not waver: your anticipatory anxiety will start to moderate. Once you commit, the internal debate stops, and without the constant attention on trying to decide one way or another—measuring risk, planning potential escape, worrying about what could happen—your anticipatory anxiety reduces and starts to take a back seat. *A solid commitment brings relief.*

This is what we mean when we say that anticipatory decreases with decision—no matter what choice you make.

HELPFUL FACT—Anticipatory anxiety increases with indecision.

Later, we will show how avoidance is precisely the way that anticipatory anxiety gets reinforced and strengthened in the longer run. But, for the moment, you can notice how anticipatory anxiety and avoidance are intertwined. Anticipatory anxiety only exists when you are actively intending to do something, go somewhere, face the source of your fear, perform, travel, or otherwise contact the source of your agony.

Now that you understand some of the ways that indecision and avoidance contribute to anticipatory anxiety, let's take a closer look at some of the ways that anticipatory anxiety manifests itself.

Five Presentations of the Anticipatory Anxiety Experience

We describe here some of the most common ways that anticipatory anxiety presents itself. You might notice that all these forms of anticipatory anxiety are inadvertently self-perpetuating. These include unhelpful attitudes, fantasies of catastrophe, experiential and behavioral avoidance, along with internal dialogues of bargaining, arguing, and planning. This is precisely why anticipatory anxiety is such a pervasive phenomenon and why it persists despite your best efforts. Many of these may initially seem like coping methods for dealing with anxiety, but in fact they backfire and keep anxiety going. In future chapters, we will address in detail why each form of anticipatory anxiety reinforces itself and provide clear directions for how to reverse this self-perpetuating process.

Intending to white-knuckle. This may be the most common presentation. You find yourself committed or obligated, and you get the automatic whoosh of fear. You remember the intense anxiety you felt last time. You say to yourself, *I can't back out of this. I will just HAVE to do it. No matter how awful I feel, I'm gonna get through this. This is going to be terrible.* Unfortunately, most of the time, this is a formula for ensuring that anticipatory anxiety wins the battle. One of two things will happen. Either, as you get closer to the actual event, your anxiety skyrockets, and you decide to cancel anyway. Or, you do go, but your experience leading up to the event is such an ordeal that, no matter how it goes or how you do, the misery of anticipation becomes vividly embedded in your memory. And your experience of anticipatory anxiety usurps the memory of the actual event, so you feel no better the next time. Plowing through the experience remains painful.

The opposite attitude to white-knuckling is the concept of willingness. Willingness is what makes it possible to build on anxious experiences toward recovery, rather than simply dreading each consecutive grueling activity. We will introduce this concept in chapter 8.

Debating whether to avoid. You are fearful of flying but decide to take a family trip to Disneyland. You become frightened as soon as the trip is planned but tell yourself that you can always back out. You let the family know that they might have to go without you. When the tickets are bought, you feel more trapped, and you have another spike in anxiety. But you still aren't entirely sure that you will make the flight. As the flight draws closer, you experience waves of anxiety imagining all the catastrophic things that might happen on your flight. You debate with yourself. *Should I go, or should*

I stay home? You decide to wait until you get to the airport before making a final decision. Now your anticipatory anxiety is really high. Your mind starts to ping-pong between *Should I fly?* and *Should I bail out now?* This internal debate continues almost incessantly, elevating your anticipatory anxiety and making it harder to commit. In extreme cases, you may still be debating with yourself as you step on the plane and fasten your seat belt. You might decide you can't do it just before the door closes and bolt off the plane, feeling much relieved of your anticipatory anxiety but also feeling like a failure for letting your anxiety take control.

Planning how to cope or escape. Someone has asked you on a dinner date. They seem attractive, but you do not know much about them. You want to go, but you are immediately both anxious and excited. So, you do your research: Google, Facebook, and Instagram searches; contact with anyone who might know the person; and advice from friends and family. As a result, you delay responding to a text from the person so you can think about it. You consider if you really have time in your life for dating. You plan eight different scripts to follow depending on what they might say. You are in a tizzy. When you finally accept the date, you decide that you will drive yourself to the restaurant so you have the option of making an excuse and leaving right away. Then you call your friend and ask her to contact you with both a text and a phone call about one hour after the date is scheduled to begin, providing a cover story in case you want to leave. When you get to the restaurant, you order a vodka martini and drink it down before your date arrives. The date goes quite well, but was it the escape planning or the vodka, or would it have been fine without these vices? Because you attribute your success to these coping mechanisms, you still believe you will need them the next time you have anticipatory anxiety and will not learn to feel comfortable without them.

Oscillating avoidance. Sometimes avoiding one source of anxiety puts you smack into contact with yet another type. This is the embodiment of the saying, "Damned if you do, and damned if you don't." Suppose you have an extreme fear of colon cancer. You schedule a routine colonoscopy, and then become overwhelmed with anticipatory anxiety, imagining that you will discover that you do, indeed, have cancer. Or that you will die of a medical error under twilight sleep. So, you cancel the screening and experience some immediate relief. However, you then imagine that your cancer is progressing through your body, and this produces another powerful surge of anticipatory anxiety. How do you avoid this one? You schedule the colonoscopy once again. Of course, this starts up yet another new round of anticipatory anxiety, avoidance, new anxious anticipation, and so on.

Trying to put it out of your mind. When you are anxious about some upcoming event, and you try to put it out of your mind, think about it later, or otherwise banish the thought from your consciousness, this is yet another way of trying to cope with anticipatory anxiety. The major problem here is that trying to push a thought out of your mind is a bit like trying to push back the tide or trying to stop the sun from setting. It just does not work. We wrote about this extensively in *Overcoming Unwanted Intrusive Thoughts* (Winston and Seif 2017). The effort you spend trying to get the worry thoughts out of your mind makes them more pronounced. This is a prime way to increase your anticipatory anxiety.

Perhaps you have already identified for yourself the way you usually try to handle anticipatory anxiety. Let's look at some examples of real people whose lives are impacted by anticipatory anxiety and whose attempts to cope are not working.

Types of Anticipatory Anxiety

All types of anticipatory anxiety share the features of unwanted feelings and the urge to avoid. But there are significant differences in how they develop.

So far, we have pointed out that anticipatory anxiety fuels the avoidance aspect of anxiety. It bothers you when you are intending to proceed, and then as soon as you choose to avoid, your anxiety plummets. Anticipatory anxiety can stem from different sources. Understanding these will help you overcome it. We've categorized anticipatory anxiety into five types, based on what the anxiety stems from, and provide an overview of each below. As we describe each type, we illustrate how it looks by presenting some real examples. The people we describe are based on real people we have known, with details changed so they remain unrecognizable.

In real life, people may have aspects of more than one kind of anticipatory anxiety and more than one kind of experience as they attempt to deal with it. In the course of a lifetime, themes may change from one focus to another, ineffective coping strategies may be adopted and then abandoned, and catastrophic thinking can change as well. As you read about the type of anticipatory anxiety and the illustrating vignettes, see if you can spot how each person has become embroiled in their own exaggerated worries and reactions and what unhelpful steps they attempt.

Imagination Based

In imagination-based anticipatory anxiety, your overactive and creative imagination can instantly conjure up scenes of catastrophic outcomes and a wide array of things that could go wrong—an amalgam of stories you have heard, unlikely but real possibilities, and a tendency toward assuming the worst even if the probability is extremely low. Media coverage of disasters, accidents, and bizarre events can heighten this type of anxiety. An example of imagination-based anticipatory anxiety is experiencing intense anxiety while imagining what a doctor might say about a mole that you already have decided is melanoma. Another example is watching the coverage of an air disaster or the victims of COVID-19 and imagining how terrifying it would be to find yourself in that situation. Yet another might be feeling anxious about driving to a new location because you imagined having difficulty finding a parking space and you are already embarrassed about arriving late. Imagination-based anticipatory anxiety is common in—but not exclusive to—people with obsessive-compulsive disorder and generalized anxiety.

A variant of imagination-based anticipatory anxiety involves a catastrophic elaboration of a real experience that could have happened but didn't. For example, you may come home and realize that you had neglected to turn off a stove burner. You feel a shock of fear and imagine your house burning down. Nothing happened, but you have now made yourself anxious even thinking about using the stove because you could have burned the house down.

WHAT IT LOOKS LIKE

John says he is insecure because he cannot even think about speaking in class without getting sweaty and feeling like he can't breathe. He never raises his hand and spends the whole time in algebra class hoping the teacher does not call on him. Sometimes he feels like he might pass out in class if he thinks the teacher is going to call on him. He imagines himself making a fool of himself in front of everyone and how he could not stand the humiliation. He wants to drop out of school.

The next example of imagination-based insomnia is a common form of anticipatory anxiety for both teens and adults. Ellery's mother recognized the pattern of insomnia that indicates the presence of anticipatory anxiety. It is Ellery's imagined school failures, none of which have ever happened, that keeps her up at night. She has no intention of avoiding school: she just hopes to avoid messing up.

Ellery's mom noticed that her daughter had trouble sleeping every Sunday night. Ellery is an excellent student but told her mom she was worried that something could happen to "break her record of all As." Perhaps there would be a pop quiz or she might not have done her assignment right. She is very nervous every Monday morning but feels more relaxed at school and sleeps well on the other nights of the week.

The following is an example of an adult who continuously imagines the worst, believes her own worries, and keeps herself in a constant state of anticipatory anxiety.

Shakira began her therapy session saying she had had a terrible week because she knew she was dying and was worried about how her children would manage and whether she could bear the ordeal that was coming. She was awaiting the results of some diagnostic blood tests, which she was sure would indicate a fatal disease. She dreaded her upcoming doctor appointment, only two days away. The following week, she sheepishly told her therapist that everything was normal—for now. But she still felt that she was suffering from some undiagnosed malady. This is an ongoing pattern in which Shakira's imagination and her feeling of anxious uncertainty about her health make it impossible to learn the simple lesson that her anticipatory anxiety is continually tricking her.

The variety of fearful images that you can conjure up when facing travel is a common source of anticipatory anxiety. In this case of imagination-based anticipatory anxiety, escape and avoidance planning play a major role in generating even more anxiety—even though it is never needed.

Jamison needs to travel out of state by car several times a month for work. The days leading up to each business trip are a horror show for him. He checks the weather reports several times a day, can't sleep the night before, and often vomits before leaving. He worries that his dog sitter will get sick and not take care of his dog, even though this has never happened. He worries about his car breaking down and has two emergency car services and a backup third one. He imagines being late due to traffic. He imagines falling asleep at the wheel. He plots the location of hospitals along the way just in case. He thinks he might be getting too old to be doing this, and then he would have to quit his job. The most extraordinary aspect of this fear is that once he is actually on the road, his anxiety is quite manageable. But it never seems to get easier before he leaves.

Here is an example of imagination-based anxiety that presents as an oscillating avoidance pattern. This often appears for those who have an exaggerated fear of physical illness. Sometimes the casual suggestion of a health professional can trigger ongoing anticipatory anxiety.

Bjorn is a healthy forty-six-year-old man and an avid runner who completed three marathons before the age of thirty-five. Now a father of two young girls, he keeps worrying about the possibility of serious illness. During a routine health exam, his physician told him that many people were now getting a baseline "calcium score" that shows the amount of calcium in the arteries of the heart—a quick, inexpensive, noninvasive test that Bjorn could get within the next few years. This simple suggestion triggered a near panic! He had never worried about his heart before—only cancer, brain tumors, and HIV. But now he was terrified that the test might show advanced levels of heart disease. Bjorn scheduled the test but was flooded with horrible anticipated results of advanced cardiac disease. He decided to cancel the test at the last minute. But he then imagined that he was about to have a heart attack and this test would be the only way to save his life. So, he rescheduled the test, only to once again cancel hours before his appointment. But of course, this cancellation created the other form of anticipatory anxiety. He felt incompetent, stuck, and unable to make any decision and worried that the stress of the anticipatory anxiety itself would result in his death by heart disease.

There is no relief with avoidance when Bjorn is caught between two different fears.

There are times when you may not even realize that your avoidances are motivated by anticipatory anxiety. You might acknowledge that you are frightened by something, but you don't quite connect your ongoing avoidance with anticipatory anxiety. The next two examples of anticipatory anxiety demonstrate avoidances that feel accidental, automatic, or even unrelated.

Sometimes avoidance manifests itself as a series of mistakes, delays, oversights, or bad luck. This patient's imagined outcomes are producing avoidance behaviors that he is not fully aware of.

Gus came to therapy because of his excessive fear of illness. He acknowledges that going to the doctor is frightening but agreed to yearly routine checkups. Despite this, he has extraordinary difficulty scheduling appointments and then getting to them once he sets them up. One time he inadvertently went to the office of his former internist! He never realized it and couldn't understand why his appointment wasn't on their calendar. Another time he was unable to operate the buzzer system to open the door. It didn't occur to him to phone the receptionist to relay the problem. It has now been three years since his last physical, and he worries that his delay may have allowed any disease to progress. Despite this, Gus has real trouble acknowledging that it is his anticipatory anxiety—rather than a spate of bad luck, poor timing, and silly mistakes—that accounts for him not making annual doctor appointments.

Gus's anticipatory anxiety showed up as inattention and errors.

> HELPFUL FACT—Anticipatory anxiety can manifest as a brain fog that results in mistakes, delays, and oversights.

The next example of an imagination-based anxiety is especially worth noting because of the nature of the distress. Sometimes anticipatory anxiety can present as a general malaise: you might feel sick right before a big event and then be quite surprised when your "illness" magically disappears after the event.

Jose took an improv class and felt totally sick before the big performance in front of a live audience. He had a headache, sore throat, and nausea, and he kept shivering. He kept taking his temperature, trying to decide if he should go, but it was normal. He almost hoped for a fever because that would settle it. His anxiety was focused on trying to decide whether he should just go anyway or stay home. He was unaware that the "sickness" was anticipatory anxiety and that it would likely subside once he got there and got involved.

Jose's anxious body was tricking him into feeling ill.

> HELPFUL FACT—Anticipatory anxiety can feel like an acute illness that magically gets better as soon as the feared event is over.

Or, anticipatory anxiety can feel like guilt or overbearing irresponsibility when imagining catastrophic changes in the future.

Sandy read an article about food insecurity that would be caused by climate change and how this would affect human global migration in the next decades. She could not sleep afterward. She kept imagining herself carrying a small hungry child on a long march through a hot dry landscape and the hunger and poverty that was sure to come. She decided she would drop out of school and dedicate her life to fighting climate change but then felt it would be irresponsible to waste her parents' money. She was having trouble with tightness in her chest and a feeling of being smothered. She feels constantly guilty when she thinks that she will likely be okay but others won't.

Here's another typical onset of imagination-based anticipatory anxiety: it is a reaction to realizing that a terrible thing could have happened even though it did not.

Hilda is an eighty-nine-year-old widow who lives independently with delivered groceries and a car service when she needs it. She is proud to cook for herself and manage her own affairs, including her investments and her minimal medical needs. Recently, however, she stumbled over a throw rug in her bathroom and fell into the shower stall, twisting an ankle. She called her daughter but refused a 911 call, hobbling around her house with a cane until she could walk unsupported. To her surprise, she can't stop thinking that she could have been seriously injured, and now she's acutely afraid of falling. She hangs on to furniture and walls and is anxious whenever she must go out. She will only wear one pair of shoes that she considers safe and sensible. Her whole attitude about going places on her own has changed even though her injuries were relatively minor. This anticipatory anxiety makes her feel old and vulnerable and embarrassed. Her thoughts of What if? make her hypervigilant, watching for another even worse mishap.

Memory Based

Memory-based anticipatory anxiety is a conditioned anxious response that occurs when you recall a previous panic attack or very high level of distress. It is less a product of imagination than a function of the memory of a vivid actual prior experience. The situation in which this distress occurred becomes associated with and connected to the anxiety. It is a conditioned response. This type of anticipatory anxiety tends to happen automatically. If you had a panic attack in an elevator—even if years ago—your memory of it can remain very vivid, and every time you contemplate taking an elevator again, anxiety is provoked. Your tendency is to recoil and become hesitant to put yourself in that situation again, as if all elevators are dangerous to you and will trigger the same intense anxiety. This may persist well after you have had many uneventful elevator rides. Memory-based anticipatory anxiety can show up as physical manifestations of anxiety even if you are not consciously aware of the connection to a past event.

Similarly, if you once froze in front of your fifth-grade class while presenting a book report, you may have echoes of that experience even in adulthood, and it may have generalized to any situation in which the spotlight of attention is on you or you are concerned about the judgment of your performance by others. Even imagining speaking up in a meeting might trigger the memory of shame and misery you experienced decades before and provoke anticipatory anxiety. This kind of anticipatory anxiety is common in panic disorder, all kinds of phobias, and social and performance anxiety.

WHAT IT LOOKS LIKE

In this example of memory-based anticipatory anxiety, debate over returning to the site of a panic attack is inadvertently fueling dread.

Myra is an independent young engineer who lives in terror of having a panic attack on a bridge. Two years ago, while driving to visit a friend who lives on the other side of the bay, she noticed a rapid heartbeat, woozy sensations, and tightness in her chest. She told herself she was just tired and kept driving, but when she got on the bridge, she suddenly realized she could not pull over if she had to and then had her first full-fledged panic attack. This experience has haunted her ever since even though it has not happened again. But she has not been on a bridge either. Now she is trapped in a commitment to visit her friend again. She is having trouble sleeping. She keeps imagining an embarrassing scene in which she does pull over on the bridge, stopping traffic, looking like a hyperventilating lunatic. She is debating making yet another excuse to avoid going.

The memory of an unpleasant experience paired with the memory of a sensation in the body can trigger memory-based anticipatory anxiety. In the example below, the sensation of feeling "full" was the trigger, but there are types of memory-based anticipatory anxieties that are associated with sights, sounds, smells, and tastes as well as with physical sensations.

Shantee has worried about vomiting since she had food poisoning when she was a little girl. After that, she sometimes refused to go to school for fear she might vomit in class. As an adult, whenever she needs to drive out of her neighborhood, she makes sure that she never eats enough to feel full because she associates the feeling of fullness in her stomach with vomiting. If she has eaten a big meal and feels full when called to drive, she waits until the feeling goes away.

Anticipatory anxiety can be generalized—as in the example of someone who fears and avoids all situations in which they might feel trapped or all situations in which they might be judged. Or it can be quite specific. Here is an elementary school student who enjoys some social events but experiences anticipatory anxiety prior to others.

Amy is a ten-year-old girl who suffers from anticipatory anxiety whenever she is about to attend a party or is part of a social gathering. Interestingly, she looks forward to going to school and enjoys playdates with one or two friends. But she stays seated in the car when she must enter a house with many people inside, and she often complains of having a "tummy ache" right before birthday parties. Her dad thinks this started when she was teased by a girl's older brother at a birthday party last year. She gets cranky and upset as the time to leave approaches, and she will sometimes just freeze at the front door of a house instead of ringing the bell or walking in with her companions.

She can't explain what bothers her. This avoidance of large groups of people occurs whether or not she is with family.

Many children like Amy cannot tell us they are experiencing anticipatory anxiety, but their actions show it. In Amy's case, her fears are likely imagination-based worries combined with memories of difficult experiences. This is not an uncommon combination.

Traumatic-Trigger Based

Traumatic-trigger-based anticipatory anxiety automatically emerges when you imagine coming into contact with an event—or series of events or reminders—that caused you great pain, anxiety, or moral injury in the past. This type of anticipatory anxiety is more reality based than imagination based; however, it is exaggerated by past experience of actual trauma. An example would be extreme anxiety about returning home for a family event where you may briefly encounter a family member who was abusive years ago. You are likely anticipating unwanted feelings at the thought of seeing them even if there is no expectation of interacting with them.

WHAT IT LOOKS LIKE

Anticipating contact with a traumatic trigger can boost ordinary discomfort to intense anticipatory anxiety. In the following example, Enzo felt "pure panic" about a school reunion. Traumatic memories amplify anticipatory anxiety for Enzo.

Enzo grew up in a lower-class section of Boston and went to parochial school, where some of his teachers were exceedingly cruel. Enzo has vivid memories of being repeatedly humiliated by one particularly nasty eighth-grade teacher and of the fear and humiliation that followed him that entire academic year. When he received an invitation to his twenty-fifth school reunion, his anticipatory anxiety spiked, but he was determined to attend. He made escape plans, including the possibility of an early exit. He decided that he would "fortify" himself with one or two drinks beforehand and made sure his wife understood that they

might suddenly leave if he actually comes into contact with the
previously offending teacher. Recently he has had nightmares in which
he is being bullied or berated by a faceless person.

Sensitivity to Expected Anxiety

As we have seen, an overactive imagination can be a powerful anxiety-creating force, especially if you are alone and your imaginings focus on the catastrophic possibilities that can bedevil you. This is especially true for people who feel vulnerable and inadequate to handling anxiety and expect themselves to "fall apart" in an emergency. Anxiety sensitivity is a general fear of anxiety or distress. It stems from beliefs about your inability to cope with the physical sensations of arousal or the psychological experience of anxiety in general, leading you to approach certain situations with a feeling of fragility. You might feel—within the context of these situations—a particularly intense sense of incompetence or inability to manage. As a result, you dread them. Often, the situations that produce this type of anticipatory anxiety involve novelty, excitement, or a particular challenge. Others might experience anxiety in these situations, but there is one big difference: you are afraid not only of the situation, but also frightened by the expected anxiety. This anxiety sensitivity comes in the form of *What if I can't stand it, or what if I can't manage or function because the anxiety overpowers me?* Past successes at navigating novelty and prior resilience seem overshadowed, explained away, or discounted.

WHAT IT LOOKS LIKE

In this example, Nia is so afraid of being afraid, so convinced that she cannot take care of herself when anxious, that she believes she cannot be alone at night.

When she learns that her husband is going to be away, Nia
immediately begins to search for one friend to be on "standby" and
another to be on "backup standby" just in case something happens and
she needs help when she is alone. She imagines falling in the shower,

getting sick, hearing strange noises outside, or perhaps the electricity going out. She comforts herself by carrying her cell phone everywhere in the house. She thought about signing up for a senior's medic alert to wear around her neck but was embarrassed because, at thirty-nine, she has no medical conditions, and her husband is already critical of her.

In another example of anxiety sensitivity-based anticipation, Natalia doubts her ability to parent in the context of her panic disorder and social anxiety. The fear of having a panic attack, a humiliating experience, or an unbearable level of anxiety feels like an insurmountable challenge. But avoidance leads to feelings of guilt and questioning about the quality of her parenting. Underlying issues of self-doubt and insecurity feed her expectations of being inadequate to the task at hand.

Natalia has a seven-year-old daughter. She and her husband immigrated from Belarus, and she speaks fluent English with an accent. Since her daughter started school, she dreads contact with the mothers of her classmates. Shy by nature and suffering from panic attacks that she tries to hide, the combination of social anxiety, embarrassment over her foreign accent, and the fear of panicking has pushed Natalia to avoid all contact with the parents of her daughter's friends. As a result, her daughter is missing out on contact with her peers and has been asking why she is the only one in her class who has no playdates.

Nia and Natalia share the trait of anxiety sensitivity—being afraid of anxiety itself. They fear the physical manifestations that occur in a panic attack or during high levels of anxiety, as well as the psychological experience of anxiety. We will explore anxiety sensitivity in more detail in chapter 3.

HELPFUL FACT—Anxiety sensitivity can be a powerful source of anticipatory anxiety.

Mood Based

Finally, mood-based anticipatory anxiety can be present during periods of clinical depression, illness, or other biologically driven mood states. For example, during a postpartum period, with changing hormones and little sleep, you may uncharacteristically feel anticipatory anxiety about seeing other people. Or if you are struggling with depression that is robbing you of enthusiasm for anything, activities you may normally look forward to can become things you dread and may provoke anticipatory anxiety. When you feel withdrawn, not yourself, unable to perform at your normal capacities, or unable to concentrate or enjoy anything, then it is natural to have anticipatory anxiety about obligations, encounters with others, and even activities you usually cherish. Treatment of the underlying condition will restore you to your usual self-confidence, and then this kind of anticipatory anxiety naturally recedes.

WHAT IT LOOKS LIKE

When feelings of intermittent depression take over, people who are usually comfortable and confident often look at every task as overwhelming and enervating. Here is an example of mood-based anticipatory anxiety. Kevin's clinical depression makes him feel withdrawn and "not himself."

Kevin has suffered from recurrent clinical depression. When he is feeling well, he is a popular, outgoing fellow, often taking leadership positions in his workplace, and usually better than most at keeping an even keel under stress. Only his wife knows about his mental health issues. Recently, his antidepressant stopped being effective, and he is switching medication. He feels slowed down, has trouble concentrating, sleeps poorly, and has lost weight. He feels worthless like this and has been barely managing to work from home since the COVID-19 pandemic began. But there will come a time when he will have to go back to the office in person, and he is dreading this. If I am like this, everyone will know there is something wrong, I don't think I can face any more work assignments, and I feel so withdrawn and nonfunctional. Even though there is no date set for him to return to the office, and there is every reason to believe his new medications will help, he has so much anticipatory anxiety that he is considering medical leave on the basis of migraines, not mental health.

HELPFUL FACT—Anticipatory anxiety can stem from imagination, memory, expected traumatic triggers, anxiety sensitivity, or mood.

These examples certainly don't illustrate the entire range of anticipatory anxieties, but they allow you to gain a sense of where and how anxious anticipation manifests as—and pushes for—avoidance.

Self Study

Learn to recognize your own anticipatory anxiety. As you look back at situations you have avoided and times you have suffered needlessly before undertaking a choice or a challenge, try to identify anticipatory anxiety. Take your time. Can you point out instances in which you did not do or could not do something you wanted to do because of it? Each day this week, contemplate circumstances in your life that provoke anticipatory anxiety. See if you can notice how indecision may play a role. And notice how avoidance or the urge to avoid takes hold.

Conclusion

So far, we've introduced the phenomenon of anticipatory anxiety, a component of almost all anxieties, and described how it is a separately identifiable component of the anxious experience. We touched on anticipatory anxiety's ability to fool you into thinking that your anxiety is a harbinger of what is in store for you. We presented our best guesstimate on how common it is. We described how anticipatory anxiety presents across the lifespan and some common ways of experiencing it. We looked at the role of indecision in inadvertently perpetuating and exacerbating anticipatory anxiety. We explored how it looks in real life. Identifying anticipatory anxiety will allow you to focus on the role of avoidance in maintaining your anxiety. Identifying how this phenomenon operates in your life will equip you to overcome the impediments that keep you from living the life you want.

CHAPTER 2

Chronic Indecisiveness: Between a Rock and a Hard Place

Chronic indecisiveness is about getting stuck at a choice point, unable to proceed. It can happen on a regular basis with small meaningless choices (*Which movie should I watch? Which brand of cereal should I buy?*) as well as with consequential choice points (*Should I marry this person? Buy this house?*). It is the habit of avoiding a decision, sometimes agonized, anxious, and conscious and sometimes unconscious. There is often a large component of anticipatory anxiety in chronic indecisiveness, and as we discussed in chapter 1, indecision often fuels and exacerbates anticipatory anxiety. Procrastinators and perfectionists are often dealing with chronic indecisiveness. So are a lot of people with obsessive-compulsive disorder (OCD). This chapter explores chronic indecisiveness in its many forms.

Here is what chronic indecisiveness can look like:

Carol had constant trouble making up her mind. When her hot water heater broke, she couldn't decide which type to get. When her oven broke, she couldn't decide between a cooktop or a range. For months her house was without a stove or hot water. Her children rarely got birthday gifts although she spent hours looking for the "right" gifts. She was chronically late to social appointments because she was never sure what outfit to wear. She wanted to move to another apartment but never seemed to find the right one despite extensive apartment hunting. Meanwhile, her family of four lived in a small two bedroom even though they could afford something larger. Carol mused over all her missed opportunities but was unable to break that cycle. Carol suffered from chronic indecisiveness.

Can you relate to Carol's experience? If you struggle with chronic indecisiveness, you may focus on the doubts you experience when you do not feel certain of the "right" decision to make. Or you may just get stuck, procrastinate, forget, or avoid because the consequences of any decision could take you down the wrong path, end in dire results, or produce regrets. Chronic indecisiveness, which is common in people with obsessive-compulsive disorder, generalized anxiety, or depression, is a habit—a style—of not making a decision. It is a way of operating in the world. Just like anticipatory anxiety, overthinking and imagination about the future play an important role in paralyzing action. In contrast to anticipatory anxiety, though, chronic indecisiveness may involve a great deal of anxiety or little or no overt or conscious anxiety.

HELPFUL FACT—Chronic indecisiveness is a recurring tendency to avoid decisions and to get stuck.

More Than Ordinary Indecision

It is entirely common to avoid making decisions—big and small—at various times in our lives. We all know people who get stuck at some point, seemingly unable to make a choice; just about everyone can identify a time they had trouble making some decision. That is normal—sometimes you just can't be sure enough or don't have information you need, so you put off a decision for a while. Getting stuck at certain choice points does not constitute chronic indecisiveness. The difference is that those who aren't chronically indecisive get unstuck and manage to get on with their lives. In contrast, chronic indecisiveness is an enduring tendency of not making decisions and getting stuck. We are talking about a general tendency, a style, of not making choices.

Some people with chronic indecisiveness seem to be unable to make decisions across the board, while others have little difficulty making choices in some aspects of their life but are paralyzed by chronic indecisiveness in others. For example, someone might be assertive and decisive at work but unable to make commitments or choices in the realm of romantic relationships. Or someone may be a confident parent day-to-day and also be utterly unable to choose a hairdresser or a vacation spot.

We are unable to provide any hard statistics about the number of people who experience chronic indecisiveness since it is not a diagnostic category and there are no valid surveys of this problem. Many people with chronic indecisiveness think of it as "just my personality," feel bad about themselves, and do not seek help. This is extremely unfortunate because there are effective ways of addressing these issues. Additionally, this type of paralysis can be an aspect of other problems—including anxiety, OCD, and depression—all of which can be treated effectively. Chronic indecisiveness is not a personality trait; it is a behavioral problem that can be changed. It also looks different from person to person, as we'll discuss next.

HELPFUL FACT—Chronic indecisiveness is not a personality trait: it is a behavioral problem that can be changed.

Four Ways of Avoiding Decisions

Each person with chronic indecisiveness has particular areas of sensitivity and individual patterns of avoiding decisions. Here are the four most common patterns of not making a choice. You might have a particular way of not choosing, and we suggest that you pay attention to your own manner of chronic indecisiveness and avoiding making choices.

Procrastinating and Delaying

While "procrastinating" refers to knowing what you need to do but being unable to just make the decision in the moment to do it, "delaying" is closer to declining to make a decision. Here is an example of procrastination.

Assad needs to submit his online college application by a specific date. He has his heart set on getting accepted by his favorite school. He is also an avid cyclist, so he plans to start the application as soon as his cycling season winds down. Yet whenever he logs on, he finds himself perusing the cycling journal pages, checking on new equipment for his bike, and imaging the pleasure his newest high-tech cycling device will bring. He is also a devoted gamer. And so, just when he starts to feel the pressure of the deadline coming close, he finds out that a brand-new version of his favorite game is being released. He can't stop playing. Finally, the night before the application is due, his parents pull the plug on the gaming, and he manages to complete the application at the very last minute. He has the same pattern with many all-nighters before tests.

In the example of delaying, Tapani is declining to make a decision.

Tapani was an enthusiastic member of Toastmasters and attended meetings to hone his sales skills. It took him years to decide to go for certification. He needed to complete twelve lunchtime mini-lectures within a six-month period to qualify. He spent the first five months unable to commit to any topic, nail down any date to talk, or consider any talk ready. He finally gave twelve mini-lectures in three weeks. This kind of delay is a pattern in his life. He took such a long time to decide between two job offers that both disappeared. When he was up for possible promotion, he delayed submitting his performance review because he could not decide how to rate himself and lost the opportunity.

Active Evasion (Head in the Sand)

Evasion is about dodging any aspects of the decision you're unwilling to make and pretending there's no decision you need to make.

Aphrodite is a successful small businesswoman and is the first in her extended family to become an entrepreneur. She has had a contentious relationship with her family for years. When she became entwined in an argument over finances with her younger sister, she ignored her sister's angry emails and didn't answer her phone calls or texts. One day she got an email from a lawyer, stating that he was retained by the sister and that she should retain a lawyer to represent herself. Still, Aphrodite didn't respond to this request. When she finally consulted a therapist, she admitted that she had over two hundred unopened emails relating to this conflict. She had been unable to decide whether to give in to her sister's demand or to stand her ground, so she just avoided the whole thing.

Forgetting

Forgetting—sometimes called "convenient forgetting"—is a way of avoiding that which is just outside of one's awareness. It may seem to be accidental, until a pattern appears.

Matthew's wife is concerned about his marijuana use, but he is ambivalent about whether he wants to stop. Some days he wants to cut back or even stop using marijuana, and some days he doesn't. He has agreed to go to therapy to address this but keeps missing his therapy appointments. He puts them in his phone calendar, but then he forgets to check his phone when he starts his workday. Then he realizes a few hours after missing his appointment that he just "forgot." He also doesn't remember the promises he makes to do his therapy homework assignments; they just fly out of his mind. He decides to go a month without using marijuana, but then forgets his promise to himself and takes a hit.

Making Decisions with Escape Clauses

Returnable, exchangeable, reversible, redo-able choices may make every potential decision a tentative one, allowing for endless deliberations without making a committed choice.

Karen has been looking for the perfect watch for two years. She buys—and then returns—one watch after the other. She only buys fully refundable watches. One watch is too garish, one too plain, one might make someone think she is showing off, one is so ordinary that no one will notice it. Sometimes the issue is whether she deserves the watch when others go hungry. Sometimes she takes it back just because she feels her purchase was too impulsive; other times, she will mull over a watch and keep looking at it online multiple times a day and never order it. She decided that watches are obsolete since everyone carries a cell phone—and then changed her mind yet again. She is still looking.

> HELPFUL FACT—Ways of being stuck include procrastinating and delaying, actively evading, forgetting, and making decisions with escape clauses.

In the course of not making a decision or a choice, people may use one or any combination of these ways of being stuck, sometimes consciously avoiding anxiety, sometimes unconsciously avoiding while in distress.

Chronic Indecisiveness May Have Different Underlying Issues

Chronic indecisiveness can arise from several different issues. Some chronic indecisiveness stems directly from anticipatory anxiety. If this is true for you, your fearful narratives about catastrophic outcomes and imagined futures may lead to feeling "frozen" or "stuck" in order to prevent failures, losses, embarrassment, or distress.

In the following sections, we present six varieties of chronic indecisiveness—avoiding potential risks, avoiding "wrong" choices, trying to make the best choice (or paralysis by analysis), trying to make the "right" choice, fear of missing out, and finally, indecisiveness that you feel is justified—along with real-life examples of how each variety affects individuals.

Remember, however, that the habit of not making a decision—of remaining stuck—can show up in virtually every aspect of your life, from choosing a greeting card to choosing a spouse, from filling out a survey to deciding on a college major, from picking a place to sit to moving to another country. So, take these descriptions as a sample and not an exhaustive list. Notice also that some people have several different ways of being stuck.

Avoiding Potential Risks

The attempt to avoid potential risks underlies one kind of chronic indecisiveness related to anticipatory anxiety. Examples include not being able to commit to a doctor's appointment or to decide to confront a challenge, undertake a project, or volunteer for a position of responsibility. You may decide and then constantly revisit your decision. You likely have an escape plan for any commitment, perhaps in the form of "text me right before and I'll see if I'm up for it" or "we'll see how I feel then" or "I might change my mind." This type of chronic indecisiveness can be extremely frustrating to friends and family, who rarely get a commitment and often have to cope with last-minute cancellations and changes of plans. You may unwittingly have a reputation for being unreliable, inconsiderate, or even selfish. Avoiding potential risk is about avoiding the anticipatory anxiety that any choice provokes.

WHAT IT LOOKS LIKE

Avoiding all risk is impossible, and an attempt to do so can result in missing an important deadline. Camila is a single mother who wants the best for her seventeen-year-old daughter Fernanda. Her indecisiveness has now led inadvertently to increased risk. Camila is seeking risk-free decisions, but they are impossible.

When Fernanda turned twelve, the pediatrician recommended a vaccine against a form of cancer in women. But to be most effective, the vaccine should be administered by age thirteen or fourteen. Camila did an enormous amount of research and saw that there were both positive and negative aspects to the vaccination. Her only motivation was to shield Fernanda from risk. But she was unable to come to a decision, despite the doctor's urging that the "benefits far outweigh the risks." Still, Camila couldn't be sure. So, she continued to put off the decision. Now, Fernanda is seventeen, so the effectiveness of the vaccine would be significantly diminished, but Camila still debates whether or not to give it to her daughter.

Avoiding the "Wrong" Choice

A second type of chronic indecisiveness that stems from anticipatory anxiety is centered around avoiding making the "wrong" choice. Examples of this include situations where you can imagine having major regrets or being trapped in an untenable situation from which there is no escape. It is about avoiding a mistake—a big one, like choosing the wrong college or life partner, or a little one, like buying a nonrefundable item of clothing you might end up not liking. Here's an example: a young single woman who wanted nothing more than to have children endlessly compared the benefits of adoption, insemination, and finding a partner who had young children. Incredibly, this went on until she reached her mid-sixties, when she finally realized it was too late. This is an example of procrastination, which we briefly introduced and will talk more about in chapter 6. An active imagination for plans that go wrong, possible catastrophic outcomes, or expectations of unbearable regret fuel this type of stuckness.

WHAT IT LOOKS LIKE

Thoughts of making the wrong choice are immobilizing for some. And when the stakes seem intolerably high, avoiding the whole issue can be a way to indefinitely delay making any choice. Alvita is frozen by imagined serious regrets over making the wrong decision.

Alvita has been living with her boyfriend for eight years. She states that they seemed perfect for each other at first, but her boyfriend began changing right after they moved in together. He became distant and uncommunicative. She first started thinking about breaking up with

him after her attempts to seek counseling were ignored—almost seven
years ago. They now live quite separate lives: they sleep in separate
rooms, rarely eat meals together, and Alvita gets annoyed when her
boyfriend spends all his free time playing video games. Alvita has
become quite health conscious. She exercises regularly, eats healthily,
and has lost some weight. In contrast, her boyfriend still orders pizzas
and remains a couch potato. Whenever Alvita thinks about breaking
up, she realizes that he is a decent person who has never treated her
meanly, is a reliable breadwinner, and is supportive of Alvita's efforts
to stay healthy. Alvita talks about her conflict with two girlfriends.
One says that she should stay with him—he can be charming and
would be a dependable father to the children she would like to have.
The other says to ditch him because she can do much better. Alvita
wonders if she is asking too much. Maybe this is what relationships are
like? She imagines being with someone and having true intimacy but is
terrified that she might be making the biggest mistake of her life if she
ends this relationship. She knows that waiting so long has given her
even less time to find someone else if she wants to have children.

Here is a man whose chronic indecisiveness is focused on not making
the wrong travel and entertainment choices.

Ben is not a travel agent or concierge but knows everything there is to
know about buying tickets for anything. The ticket must be the product
of extensive research about all itinerary possibilities, mileage programs,
and every option that exists for entertainment or activities. It must be
the best deal—and he goes through a comprehensive coupon search to
make sure. The tickets must also be refundable in case he can't go or
something goes wrong. Then he repeatedly checks the weather, the
political situation, the online reviews, any new pop-up options or
opportunities, and whether he has a good or bad feeling. Last-minute
changes and cancellations are common.

This is an excellent example of someone who makes decisions with
escape clauses. For many with chronic indecisiveness, something that
seems small, like going out to dinner, can be an ordeal. How can one be

expected to choose one entrée when there might be more tasty items on the menu? Plus, there is the embarrassment of always saying, "Let the others order first, I'm still making up my mind."

Gabriella never liked to go out to eat with her friends because she was often the last person to decide what she wanted. She was overwhelmed with the choices and could never be sure what meal she wanted most. But then she solved the problem: rather than trying to decide what she wants to eat, she consciously avoids that decision and always orders the same item each time she eats out. It might not be what she wants to eat, but it saves her from the distress of having to make a decision.

Gabriella is creatively and consciously avoiding making decisions. She is sacrificing variety to prevent anxiety, much like her colleague who wears the same outfit every day (khaki pants and a white shirt) "to make things easy."

Making the Best Choice, or Paralysis by Analysis

There are also forms of chronic indecisiveness that are less driven by anticipatory anxiety. One example centers around making the best choice. This is sometimes called "paralysis by analysis." It involves having an inordinately difficult time making a choice between or among alternatives.

If you have this form of chronic indecisiveness, you go back and forth and back and forth, and nothing stands out as the one to choose. You may often do endless research, collect others' opinions, and make useless pros and cons lists. This is part of wanting to make the best choice and is related to perfectionism, which we address in chapter 6.

WHAT IT LOOKS LIKE

Here is a case of chronic indecisiveness in which a man cannot make a simple purchase, even while freely acknowledging that it doesn't matter all that much whether or not he buys the object. What is important is that he makes the best choice and not wish he had bought something else.

David has wanted to buy an aquarium for years. He can't decide whether he wants a five-gallon or a fifty-gallon one, an upright or an oblong one, fresh or saltwater fish, live or plastic plants, an expensive outlay at the beginning or to start small and build up. So far, he hasn't bought anything. The hitch is this: once he gets fish, they are living things, and he can't return them, he can't do anything but the best for them, and he might regret the purchase. He has been in and out of stores and wandering around multiple internet sites. It has not happened yet, but he believes he will know it when he sees it. Meanwhile he tells himself it doesn't really matter. His wife is sick and tired of hearing about it. For David, the desire to make the best choice results in no choice.

There are many forms of chronic indecisiveness that consist of thinking about doing something. Have you thought about volunteering at church but never actually done it? Or thought about asking out the person who sits next to you in class? Or thought about inviting a neighbor to take a walk with you? Or even thought about asking for a raise?

Sometimes thinking about doing something can also involve doing research and talking about it with other people. The distinction between chronic indecisiveness and the normal path toward activity is that in chronic indecisiveness, there is no progression to action. The person is stuck in the thinking about, the researching about, or the talking about. It doesn't matter because the end result is still inaction. No amount of discussion, thinking, or research results in an actional decision. Too much thinking is not solved by more thinking.

HELPFUL FACT—Excessive thinking about, talking about, or researching a topic is often a sign of chronic indecisiveness in the form of paralysis by analysis.

Making the "Right" Choice

Underlying another form of chronic indecisiveness is wanting to make the "right" choice. You might have an idea in your head of what you want or feel that you will know it when you come across what you want. You might shop for the right house, the right automobile at the right price, or the right *objet d'art* to fill that space in your living room. However, your efforts are often to no avail. You are waiting for that feeling of "Aha! This is it!" You are seeking a feeling of knowing for sure, or at least an absence of any doubts. While anticipatory anxiety plays a role here, this is more often related to intolerance of uncertainty (or OCD doubting), which we will be looking at in more detail in chapter 6.

WHAT IT LOOKS LIKE

When focused on being certain that you are making the right choice, what might seem like a simple choice can become overwhelming. In the end, you may lose options as others decide for you. Here is an example:

Fatima has bought a new condominium and needs to sell her old one. She bought the new condo from a real estate agent friend but has reservations about using this friend to sell her old one. She prefers choosing someone who is more established and has a more professional standing in her town but does not want to offend her friend. Unable to make the decision, she simply puts the matter out of her mind, consciously avoiding addressing the issue. The old condo stays empty for months while her husband becomes increasingly frustrated with her lack of action. Finally, the agent-friend contacts Fatima and informs her that she should put her property on the market, and she (the friend) will start showing it the following week. Fatima agrees but is still wondering if that is the right choice.

Here is an example of utter stuckness in a relationship because both people have been waiting to make the right choice for years now. They are looking for the right time to propose, and it is not happening.

PJ and her girlfriend, Linda, have been living together for eleven years. They bought a house together, they share a beloved dog, and everyone knows them as a couple. Once it became legal for them to marry, they both were elated. They talk endlessly about where they might honeymoon. PJ says that they will be together forever and is waiting until her promotion comes through before they get married. Linda is heavily involved in her own home business and is sure that they will marry once she starts to show a profit. However, neither has formally proposed, and there is no date for the wedding. They are protecting each other and themselves from the feeling of being trapped in a decision that will descend on them once a date is set. The paralysis is because they are trying to make the very best choice—not of whom to marry, but when.

Fear of Missing Out

Yet another type of chronic indecisiveness stems from a fear of missing out (FOMO)—wanting to follow all opportunities, keep all options and pathways open, and never close any doors. FOMO-motivated chronic indecisiveness concerns not making a choice because of a profound sense that making one choice precludes the alternative. FOMO can show up as being unable to choose one professional path because it closes up others or being unable to settle down with one plan of action because it means giving up another equally attractive choice. FOMO can lead to exhausting overscheduling in order to avoid making the decision to turn down any potentially exciting experience. Or the fear of not having the color of a purse you might need at some point can lead to being unable to reject any option and buying every color available. Unlike an approach-avoidance conflict (you want something, but it scares you), it is an approach-approach conflict (you want everything, but it is impossible).

WHAT IT LOOKS LIKE

The average cost of a college application is more than $50 (Kerr 2020). Colleges say that part of the reason for such a high fee is to make sure that only serious applicants apply. But look what happens when a multitude of colleges look good, and you are afraid of not applying to the one that is best for you. This is a case of FOMO.

Royce is a solid B-plus high school senior and wants to major in the arts or business. There are an enormous number of colleges that can provide a fine education for Royce, but he can't seem to narrow down his choices. Every time he researches a college, he finds at least one aspect that he definitely wants in his college education. It seems each choice has something unique to offer. His counselor tells him to apply to a maximum of ten colleges, including three that seem safe. But Royce has been unable to limit his choices, worrying that he might be missing the one that is best for him. Royce finally applied to fifty-three colleges, with a total application fee of over $3500!

Cindy also suffers from a fear of missing out:

Cindy has signed up for six different dating apps because she does not want to miss meeting the right person. She is spending hours every night scrolling through all her choices, reading everyone's profiles, and responding to dozens of text messages when she should be sleeping. She is having trouble keeping everyone straight and is completely overwhelmed. She has not actually made a date with anyone because she is too busy.

Justified Indecisiveness

Finally, we should note that there are some people with chronic indecisiveness who do not experience any conscious anticipatory anxiety. They may feel justified in continuing to do their research and delay their decisions. They may see themselves as appropriately cautious, and they may also see others who make decisions easily as too impulsive or cavalier. They may value "getting it right" as a virtue, no matter how long it takes. They are willing to suffer the frustrations of others as well as the negative effects of their inaction. These folks are unlikely to be reading this book or seeking help for their problem because it is not experienced as distressing, embarrassing, or anxiety producing. However, family and loved ones might be reading this book to help cope with or understand them.

WHAT IT LOOKS LIKE

Sometimes people justify being stuck making a decision by claiming to themselves and to others that they don't like or don't want or don't care about something. This justification tends to ring hollow to others.

Antwon still owns an old-fashioned flip phone. He claims he does not like technology or the companies that make it, but he is constantly borrowing everyone else's smartphone to search for things or look up directions. He is not able to admit how much technology he is already using despite his stated aversion to it. He would like to think this is a matter of principle and even claims that he doesn't mind texting with the old three-clicks-per-letter method. He feels justified in holding back from this purchase.

Here is another example of justified indecisiveness:

It is obvious to everyone who knows her that Cymbria wants a dog. She talks endlessly about dog choices—rescue versus purebred, long-haired versus short-haired, miniatures versus full size. She can't get through a walk in the park without stopping to pet dogs. She says she will get one when she is ready. Sometimes ready means a larger apartment. Sometimes it means having vacation time available to train the dog. Sometimes ready means having more savings. But ready never comes.

Partial Blindness: Costs of Inaction Are Often Ignored

One common aspect of chronic indecisiveness is partial blindness to the costs of inaction. In other words, you might become so preoccupied by imagining the possible negative consequences of taking the wrong action or so focused on trying to find the right action that you overlook the losses involved by taking no action. In these cases, imagining regret about an action is more powerful than realizing the actual effects of inaction. These costs include losing windows of opportunity; remaining stuck in unsatisfying circumstances; being left behind by peers, friends, and family; disappointing others; and engendering self-criticism and embarrassment.

Anticipatory worry about making a decision often starts with "What if?" Being stuck and feeling unable to act is based on the attempt to avoid that "If only..." feeling, wishing you had done something different. The sense is that the action will somehow produce regret. As a result, doing nothing feels safer. Because inaction feels like it is part of a temporarily unresolved situation (one with the potential for turning out "right"), judging the consequences of inaction along the way is delayed and not taken into account.

Another potential consequence of chronic indecisiveness may not be immediately obvious. This is how others tend to interpret your frustrating behavior—whether they let you know or are supportive. You may be perceived as selfish, inconsiderate, stubborn, unreliable, or immature. One patient was shocked when her cousin accused her of being selfish and self-centered. The cousin complained that the patient frequently changes plans last minute, makes her wait while taking an enormous amount of time to get dressed, often refuses to commit to plans, and 90 percent of the time cancels the few she makes. The patient—who is a kind and empathic person—had no idea her inability to make decisions was viewed this way.

> HELPFUL FACT—When you are paralyzed by indecisiveness, you often overlook the costs of inaction.

Self Study

Now that you are familiar with the different types of chronic indecisiveness, which of the descriptions do you identify with? Can you point out instances in your life in which you did not do or could not do something you wanted to do because of the chronic indecisiveness you experience? How do you feel about these experiences? Make a list of some areas in your life where you currently feel stuck.

Conclusion

In this chapter, we introduced you to chronic indecisiveness, five typical ways of avoiding decisions, and six main issues that underlie how people with chronic indecisiveness get stuck. We have shown you a wide range of examples of how they look in real life. Ultimately, chronic indecisiveness is a tendency—a habit—of not making decisions and thus getting stuck in certain aspects of your life. Like anticipatory anxiety, it produces avoidance. Identifying how these patterns operate in your life will equip you to overcome the impediments that keep you from living the life you want.

In the next chapter, we focus on the biological origins of anticipatory anxiety: how our brains are primed for it at birth and how our minds ultimately become stuck on the things that trigger our alarm response.

CHAPTER 3

The Biology of Anxious Bodies and Sticky Minds

In this chapter we examine how anticipatory anxiety starts and the biological and environmental factors that contribute to it. We are going to examine the role of the amygdala and how brain circuitry sets off the fight-flight-freeze response when we are faced with apparent danger. We'll also look at the inherited predispositions toward the trait of anxiety sensitivity and the experience of "sticky mind"—a term we use for a tendency to get mired in worry and get caught in looping thinking. We will also look at the way a stressful environment affects these biological underpinnings.

How Your Brain Creates Anticipatory Anxiety

We were all born without anticipatory anxiety. Newborn babies don't know that they should avoid anything. They don't envision what can happen and can't imagine what is next. But soon, as patterns form, they begin to develop expectations: when Mom picks me up, milk is on the way. We begin to anticipate what is coming. And because all creatures need the capacity to avoid real dangers to survive, we develop the capacity to imagine danger. The imaginations of children soon develop scary people, bogeymen, and monsters in the dark. As we learn more about bad things that could happen, we begin to fear strangers, going to bed at night, and dark places. We touch a hot pot and develop a memory of feeling pain, so we avoid pots, or stoves, or even kitchens. As we develop more mature emotional experiences, we learn to fear—and try to avoid—embarrassment, anger, rejection, shame, disgust, and making mistakes.

Memories of painful, overwhelming, or upsetting experiences—as well as our imaginative formulations of possible dangers—are called "triggers," and they play an essential part in the creation and maintenance of anticipatory anxiety and most chronic indecisiveness. Triggers can come in the form of a thought, an image, a feeling, or a sensation. Seeing or hearing something in the real world (a movie, a conversation, a reminder) can provoke a trigger from a memory ("I hear a baby crying and remember having had a scary thought about a baby"), or a trigger can arise during reverie before sleep ("I lie down and suddenly notice my heart beating"). It can be something real that becomes a trigger—like an elevator if you are afraid of them, a spider, a wrong turn, or a choice that needs to be made. Alternatively, it can be something entirely in the mind, like an intrusive thought or a worry about something that has never happened.

It Starts with a Trigger

Anticipatory anxiety starts with a trigger, which then results in a whoosh of upsetting emotion. While this feeling is most often anxiety or terror, it can also include the feelings of disgust, anger, shame, regret, humiliation, or any other unwanted, unacceptable, or seemingly intolerable emotion.

Here is a diagram that shows how this initial reaction is experienced.

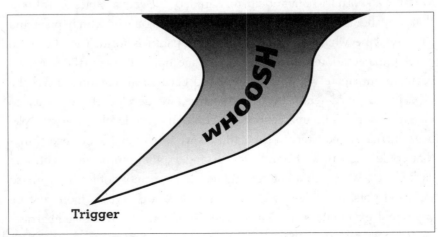

The Whoosh of Automatic Arousal

The trigger creates a rapid "whoosh" of emotion—most often fear or anxiety, but really any sort of uncomfortable or negative emotion that feels too difficult to tolerate.

> HELPFUL FACT—A trigger can be in the form of a thought, an image, a memory, or a sensation.

The Role of the Amygdala

The part of your brain that sets off this whoosh of emotion is called the "amygdala," an organ that is part of your limbic system. You can think of the limbic system as the feeling and reacting part of your brain (in contrast to the thinking part of your brain, which we will address shortly; Rajmohan and Mohandas 2007).

Your amygdala (and certain structures of your brain that surround it) can be thought of as the alarm center of your brain. It has the evolutionary purpose of warning you when you are in danger and then preparing your body and mind to respond to this threat: this is the fight-flight-freeze response that you have almost certainly heard about.

One essential aspect of the amygdala is that it is not a thinking structure of your brain. The amygdala learns by paired associations and not through rational refutation, logic, or reassurance. When you read this book, the words and ideas are talking to your cortex, not your amygdala. Creating a change in your amygdala and alarm response requires experiencing new associations and then practicing them until they become well learned. This means that you can never talk yourself out of your "whoosh" just as you can't talk yourself out of feeling angry or hungry. And just as you can't learn a new language by reading about it or how to play the piano by reading a book, changing your anticipatory anxiety will require practicing new associations as a result of having new experiences.

Your amygdala can't evaluate, ascertain, determine probabilities, or engage in any of the executive functions of the prefrontal cortex, which is the thinking part of the brain. It can't say "probably," "almost certainly," or "hardly possible at all." It can only say yes or no. There is no subtlety. This is the result of translating a world of possibilities and probabilities into a binary alarm system: The alarm can either be off or it can be on. Either the fear circuits of the brain are activated or they are not.

Remember that your amygdala's evolutionary function is to protect you from danger—to help you survive and live to pass on your DNA to the next generation. For that reason, the amygdala will sound the alarm at the merest hint of a danger: there are no survival disadvantages of sounding a false alarm. The worst that happens is that you unnecessarily prepare yourself for fight, flight, or freeze. But if your amygdala fails to warn you of a real danger, the results could be disastrous. *In other words, your amygdala operates on the principle that it is less important to find lunch right now than it is to make sure you do not become lunch right now.*

As a result, your amygdala sends out lots of false alarms. In fact, the majority of alarm signals are false. Even more relevant to anxiety, the alarms, unlike in prehistoric days, are issued not only for possible physical dangers, such as saber-toothed tigers stalking you, but for possible unwanted thoughts or feelings, disapproval, rejection, failure, or loss. Fortunately, there are ways to learn to evaluate the false alarm signals. We are going to show you how to do this. But first, let's look at the overall process.

Triggering the Amygdala

Whenever you perceive a trigger, it is picked up by a part of your brain called the "thalamus"—a kind of incoming data way station—which then immediately relays it to your amygdala. This happens extremely quickly, in less than one-fifth of a second. (This is briefer than a blink of the eye!) Speed is important because you want to be prepared for any danger as soon as possible. Fortunately, the route from the thalamus to the amygdala is direct and bypasses any of the higher brain functions. (The area of this direct route is sometimes called the "reptilian brain.")

Claire Weekes, a groundbreaking neuroscientist and author of many self-help books, used the term "first fear" (Hoare 2019) to describe this kind of automatic response to a trigger. It is key to understanding that the primitive part of your brain is outside of your conscious control. This alarm has nothing to do with willpower or intentionality. No matter how hard you try and no matter how much willpower you put into your effort, you simply cannot stop this whoosh of arousal. It just happens. It is not up to you.

The next figure demonstrates how this trigger stimulates your alarm system and the resultant alarm response.

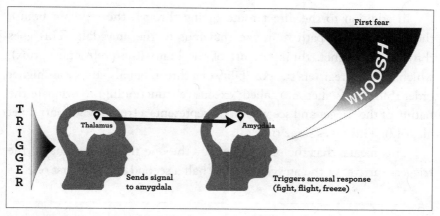

First Fear: From Trigger to Whoosh

Here are concrete examples of the automatic warning and response happening: You start to cross the street, notice a car bearing down on you, and immediately jump backward to the safety of a sidewalk. Another example: You are walking down the street and hear a loud sound. You feel a whoosh of fear as your amygdala sounds the alarm. Again, your alarm system is immediately engaged. You are primed to fight, flee, or freeze.

There is an important difference in these two examples. In the first one, your immediate response to the alarm just might have saved your life. This is a true alarm triggered by your amygdala. But the second example is different. It could be a false alarm, but you can't know that instantly. Is the loud noise a car backfiring, a firecracker, or a gunshot? Should you run, fight, or drop to the ground? Or just ignore the sound and continue onward? If it's a harmless car backfire, then the amygdala will have sent out a false alarm. But your emergency response can't wait to make that determination. After all, gunshots require immediate action. So you feel an instant whoosh whether the alarm was true or false.

Fortunately, your brain is wired to help you figure this out—it just happens a second or two after your body has reacted. We will explain that next

Two Paths to the Amygdala

In addition to the direct route (going through the reptilian brain), there is a second path from the thalamus to the amygdala. This goes through the higher, thinking part of the brain (the prefrontal cortex), which not only registers the possibility of a threat, but also uses your higher order thinking (sometimes called "executive" functioning) to evaluate the nature of the trigger and see whether it represents a true threat (Garrido et al. 2012). This takes some time.

This means that the second signal—the one that has evaluated the trigger—arrives at the amygdala about half a second *after* the first one.

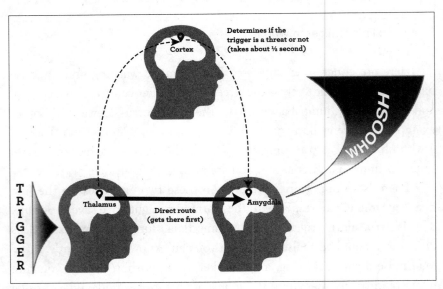

Two Paths to the Amygdala

Let's return to our previous examples: In the first case, you notice a car and jump out of the way. *This occurs prior to any thinking.* It is a reflexive part of your flight-flight-freeze reaction. Then, one-half second after your amygdala was first triggered, the message from your prefrontal cortex arrives and says something like, "That was the right response. That car could have killed you if you were hit." You may still feel shaky, and your heart might still beat fast from the adrenaline surge for a short while, but gradually you become less aroused and begin to calm down.

In the second example, your prefrontal cortex might determine that the alarm was false: "That was a car backfiring; you were in no danger. You can calm down." However, messages from your prefrontal cortex can also create a bunch of other problems—it's the way our brains create anxiety and make us feel like we are in danger when we are safe. Let's see how this happens.

You Can Be Triggered by Your Thoughts

In these two examples, suppose, after you are home and safe, your prefrontal cortex starts *imagining* what might have happened if you had failed to notice the car. It might think, *You might have been killed! What if you hadn't gotten out of the way? What if next time you don't notice the car?* These thoughts can retrigger your amygdala, and you can start to feel alarmed once again. This time, however, the triggers that set off your alarm are your thoughts—your own active imagination. If you take these thoughts reasonably seriously, you might become more cautious about crossing streets.

But if you take them too seriously—if you let your imagination hijack you—you might become so fearful of crossing streets that you start to avoid them. *You will have developed anticipatory anxiety about crossing streets!* We can diagram this in the following manner.

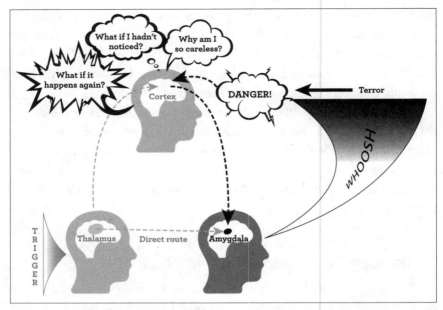

The Prefrontal Cortex Generates Anticipatory Anxiety

Now let's look at the second example—the loud noise that you heard. The sound immediately triggered you, and you felt a whoosh of arousal. Then, a half second later, you got the "all clear—just a backfire" signal. You start to relax and, in a minute or two, it's as if it never happened.

However, suppose your prefrontal cortex had determined that the sound was something you couldn't know for sure, perhaps a gunshot! Your thinking brain told you, "Your life could be in danger; take cover; you could be hurt at any time." This time, your amygdala would continue sounding the alarm. You would be heavily into your fight-flight-freeze reaction; you might run, hide, or even panic. Even though you may never really have been in danger, you were certainly afraid. The next time you think about walking down the street, this experience can haunt you, and the memory of the panic can retrigger your alarm.

Here is the lesson: Your reptilian brain is the part that first transmits the trigger to your amygdala. There is no thinking, no assessment, no subtlety, and no willpower involved. It is an automatic circuit in your brain. You cannot control this first whoosh of arousal. However, from that point onward, if your prefrontal cortex determines there is, or could be, ongoing danger—*legitimate or not*—your amygdala will continue to sound the alarm.

Your what-if thoughts can trigger your alarm system when they are spurred on by some combination of imagination, memories, mood, and sensitivity to anticipated anxiety. In general, mental images are even more anxiety triggering than word thoughts (Freeston et al. 1996).

The next figure illustrates how the what-if thought, memory, or image acts as a trigger.

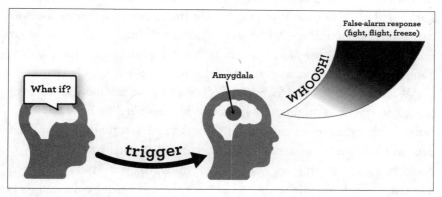

What-If Thoughts Can Trigger the Alarm Response

HELPFUL FACT—What-if thoughts can trigger your alarm system just like an external danger.

Fear and Anxiety Are Not the Same Thing

If there is a genuine external threat to our well-being, we call that reaction "fear." ("I see a mountain lion and must get away—I am afraid.") If the threat is internal—and your alarm is triggered by your imagination or memory—that is a false alarm, and we call that reaction "anxiety." ("What if I lose control and make a fool of myself? I am anxious.") The feelings may seem identical, but *you are not in danger when you are anxious.*

That's why anxiety is such a trickster—and why anticipatory anxiety is the trickiest part of anxiety. It makes you feel like you are in danger when you are safe. It is also why anticipatory anxiety provokes such powerful avoidance. You feel like you are avoiding a danger, but you are actually avoiding uncomfortable, unpleasant, or seemingly overwhelming emotions.

The physical sensations of arousal due to false alarms are your body's natural emergency-response system. They are certainly not dangerous. Despite this fact, some people hold the erroneous belief that the rapid heart rate and changed breathing from your alarm response are somehow harmful. This is untrue. If the fight-flight-freeze emergency response was dangerous (which it is not!), it would certainly be a huge design flaw in our body's evolution! Your alarm system is falsely signaling external physical danger, and you are reacting to it as if this danger is real.

What's more, much of what will allow you to overcome your anxiety hinges on the understanding that there is also no need to avoid *any* emotions or thoughts, even distressing ones. You may actually believe that certain emotional experiences are dangerous. You might think that you could not stand it, you would lose "everything," or you would fall apart. The false belief that distressing feelings or thoughts can be dangerous is often generated by prior experiences and needs to be understood, addressed, challenged, and corrected.

HELPFUL FACT—The belief that thoughts and feelings themselves can be dangerous is a false belief.

Biological Factors That Influence Anticipatory Anxiety

There are several factors that determine your own particular reactivity to false alarms. Let's begin to tease apart some of the biological factors that influence your experience of anticipatory anxiety.

Anxiety Sensitivity

In chapter 1, we noted that there are some types of anticipatory anxiety that stem from an exaggerated fear of certain bodily sensations or feelings. Psychologists call this trait "anxiety sensitivity," which is a well-researched genetic predisposition. Anxiety sensitivity consists of the tendency to fear normal bodily sensations of arousal as well as the mental and emotional experience of anxiety. Simply put, it is being afraid of fear. It can be an enduring trait—and is often accompanied by the tendency to avoid anxiety-producing situations and to worry about becoming anxious. It therefore creates a tendency toward increased anticipatory anxiety. It runs in families and is passed on by biological inheritance as well as through the messages about risk and danger in the world that you receive as you are growing up.

It is important to note that, while anxiety sensitivity is passed down both through genetics and learning, it can be substantially changed with new learning and proper treatment. Once you understand how anxiety sensitivity works, the pathway toward recovery reveals itself. In fact, one reliable measure of recovery from anticipatory anxiety is the reduction of anxiety sensitivity (Helbig-Lang et al. 2012). That is why we go into such detail here.

The following figure shows how the misinterpretation of a sensation as dangerous can continue to trigger your alarm system. This illustrates the neurological mechanism of people who have high anxiety sensitivity and how they tend to chronically fear all sensations associated with anxious arousal. The result is increased anticipatory anxiety triggered by a feared sensation.

In this illustration, we call the whoosh of arousal "second fear" (Weekes 1969) because it is created by your frightening misinterpretation of bodily sensations—the belief that you might not be able to stand it or even survive.

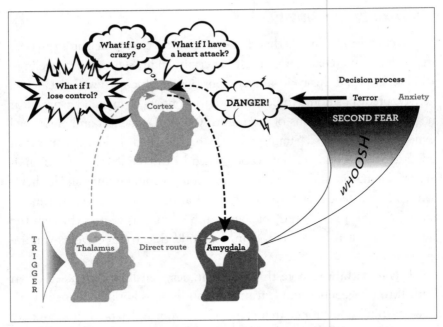

Second Fear: A Neurological Illustration of Anxiety Sensitivity

Stickiness of the Mind

Another biological factor that impacts anticipatory anxiety and chronic indecisiveness is the biological phenomenon we call "stickiness of the mind."

We use the term "stickiness of the mind" to describe the trait that is experienced as repetitive looping thinking, a sense of getting mired in worry, a talent for imaginative flights into catastrophic images and thoughts, and a tendency for junk channels of the mind to get loud and insistent instead of simply flowing by. Since it tends to run in families, you are more likely to experience this if you have a parent, grandparent, sibling, aunt, or uncle who also has a sticky mind. But stickiness is not a sign of mental illness or that something is "wrong" with you: it is a characteristic that, once understood, can be incorporated into a full and meaningful life.

The anterior cingulate cortex, a tiny brain structure, operates as a bridge between the prefrontal cortex and the amygdala. This part of the brain seems to trigger quirky, looping, repeating worry responses in people who have this predisposition to stickiness (Straube et al. 2009).

Stickiness tends to make thoughts seem important even when they are not and to demand attention and response to the inner workings of your mind when no response is really needed. Ultimately, the most effective way to live with a sticky mind is to change your relationship with your mind. This means taking a broader view, a more mindful view, a step back, or an attitude of curiosity and humor instead of judgment, alarm, and urgency. You will learn how to identify your sticky thoughts, label them as such, and realize they are not emergencies, warnings, or signals.

A sticky mind plays an important role in the creation of both anticipatory anxiety and chronic indecisiveness. When sticky thoughts are taken too seriously, it creates a reluctance to take any risks at all and a tendency to avoid triggering worries or anxious experiences. The result is that the avoidance part of anxiety (anticipatory anxiety) comes to the fore, and making decisions—both big and small—can become laborious. This sense of feeling stuck leads to limitations in living and feelings of danger, frailty, disability, and profound distress.

Stickiness of the mind is an enduring trait but, once understood, it can take its proper place and lose its ability to make you miserable.

How Stress Affects Anticipatory Anxiety

There is a complicated relationship between stress and both anticipatory anxiety and chronic indecisiveness. In general, if you're experiencing stress, that will increase the intensity of the symptoms of anxiety you feel, as well as the likelihood that thoughts and sensations can become triggers and set off false alarms. The stress response of the body can in turn increase a sense of urgency, bring on physical tension, change the way you breathe, and interfere with concentration and focus. You might have a stronger urge to avoid and have decidedly more difficulty making decisions when you are under stress.

However—and this is an essential point—stress does not cause anticipatory anxiety. Even if you could somehow reduce your stress to zero (which is not possible), you would still have difficulty making decisions and experience the desire to avoid. Avoiding stress is not the answer to overcoming anticipatory anxiety. In fact, it becomes another form of avoidance that undermines your chances to live a flexible life and develop confidence in the face of challenges. To reiterate: while it is true that all forms of anxiety are stress-sensitive, they are not caused by stress.

Avoiding stress is often the unhelpful rationalization for backing out of anxiety-producing activities or choices. Anxious arousal itself is not stress, is not dangerous, and does not need to be avoided. Avoiding anticipatory anxiety is not stress management. Taking the time and effort to understand how your imagination gets hijacked, learning a new attitude to take toward anxious arousal, and developing a new relationship with your own anxiety is the way forward.

> HELPFUL FACT—Avoiding anticipatory anxiety is not stress management.

In addition, when you are under stress, stickiness of the mind also increases. When you are tired, have a cold, are premenstrual, or drank too much last night, your thoughts may be stickier. Your mind's stickiness can also be worse when you are very hungry, lonely, angry about something, or working too hard and not sleeping much. And sometimes it's just not clear why some days are stickier than others. Whatever their cause, because sticky thoughts repeat, hang around, and keep coming back, they seem more true, more important, more urgent, and more demanding of attention. This is, of course, an illusion, but it can certainly increase the difficulty in addressing your anticipatory anxiety and rob you of confidence in making decisions.

Knowing that you are more sensitized at a particular moment can help you understand what is happening. It can help you remember that your sense of danger is exaggerated and that your feelings and thoughts are not facts or accurate predictions merely because they are strong, repetitive, loud, and sticky.

How Real-Life Events Affect Anticipatory Anxiety

Experiences in your own life, as well as events you learn about through media or conversations with others, can increase your reactivity to some what-if thoughts and make you more likely to focus on doubts and worries, feel more vulnerable, and hesitate to make decisions. A personal crisis, an ongoing ordeal, or a tragedy will understandably cause increased sensitization for a period of time. When illusions of safety or predictability have been shattered, everything may seem riskier. When you are dealing with illness, unemployment, poverty, or discrimination—the loss of real security—it is normal to feel more uncertain and to worry about real as well as imagined or potential problems.

Not allowing yourself to become hijacked by your imagination and staying focused on your own practical immediate realities may be even more important under real-world stress. Media coverage of infrequent but very dramatic events, such as terrorist attacks or collapsed bridges, may be allowed to "count" too much in evaluating your own personal safety. Hearing about someone else having an unpredicted heart attack or encountering an unusual circumstance or negative outcome does not change your own reality, but if you have a sticky mind, there is a tendency to treat these events as a new personal worry.

Your Values and Anticipatory Anxiety

The intensity of your anticipatory anxiety and your difficulties in making decisions are affected by how much the anticipated action or choice matters to you. If the outcome of an event is not so important to you, you are less likely to engage in flights of imagination about bad things happening and less likely to worry about regrets. The more casual you are about the effects of your choices, the less you agonize over making those choices.

But as something becomes more valued or important to you, anticipatory anxiety rises as well. The higher the personal stakes, the stickier the mind and the greater the anxiety. For example, there will be greater anticipatory anxiety before a job interview for a position you really desire and much less if you have other offers or don't really want the job. If generosity is an important value for you, decisions about how much to give to particular charities may be difficult or even avoided, while decisions about other expenditures may be relatively easy. Or, if you despise causing harm of any kind because kindness is a value you cherish, interactions with vulnerable people or those for whom you are responsible may provoke more anticipatory anxiety than that which is provoked when you're dealing with others.

Self Study

1. You now know that some parts of the anticipatory anxiety experiences are automatic brain processes outside your conscious control, while other parts are much more modifiable. Pick one time you experienced anticipatory anxiety and try to identify both parts of the process: what was and what was not outside of your control.

2. Evaluate your own level of anxiety sensitivity. A measure of anxiety sensitivity called the Anxiety Sensitivity Index (ASI) includes items such as the following: It scares me when my heart beats rapidly. When my chest feels tight, I get scared that I won't be able to breathe properly. When I have trouble thinking clearly, I worry that there is something wrong with me. Other items revolve around fears of embarrassment, feelings of fright caused by skipping heartbeats or pains in your chest, concerns about sweating or blushing in front of others, and fears of going crazy. What are your anxiety sensitivity fears?

3. Make note of the times in your life when you have a stickier mind and see if you can detect a pattern.

Conclusion

We have seen how the brain's normal fear circuitry can create unwarranted feelings of danger directly from certain thoughts, sensations, memories, and imagination. We also looked at the traits of both anxiety sensitivity and sticky mind, noting how both increase the experience of anticipatory anxiety and chronic indecisiveness. Additionally, the environmental stresses that add to anxiety were discussed.

In the next chapter, we look at the important role that avoidance plays. Avoidance is a natural protective behavioral response to impending danger, but when it is a response to worry, negative emotions, or feelings that seem intolerable, as opposed to actual danger, it backfires and creates more anticipatory anxiety.

CHAPTER 4

Avoidance: How Anticipatory Anxiety and Chronic Indecisiveness Get Stuck

In chapters 1 and 2, we defined anticipatory anxiety as the avoidance layer of anxiety. And we defined chronic indecisiveness as a habit of not choosing—of avoiding decisions and remaining stuck. Anticipatory anxiety is a powerful motivator for avoidance by guiding you to focus on the negative things that might happen, often with catastrophic predictions about an event. In this chapter, we explain why avoidance is such a potent engine in the generation, maintenance, and reinforcement of anticipatory anxiety. In short, catastrophic predictions lead to incapacitating anxiety and the intense desire to avoid—to keep yourself from feeling the experience of anxiety or some other uncomfortable, unpleasant emotion, sensation, or thought. And so, stopping avoidance is an essential step to gaining access to the freedom you seek. You will also learn the various manifestations of avoidance, including ways of avoiding that are not obvious at all. This is essential because you will need to understand how you avoid in order to learn how to respond differently.

Since avoidance plays such a major role in energizing and maintaining anticipatory anxiety and chronic indecisiveness, we are going to look at the myriad ways that avoidance can become part of your life. Avoidances range from the obvious—both to yourself and to others—to the subtle and hard to find. Ultimately, whatever your specific type of avoidance—whether it's through avoidance behaviors (things you do or don't do) or experiential avoidance (what you think or feel when anxiety arises)—identifying how you avoid is the first step toward recovery.

Behavioral Avoidance

A behavioral avoidance is avoidance that takes the form of an action or an inaction, usually perceptible to others, like delaying a decision or refusing to make a choice. It can be deliberate and planned, such as canceling an appointment, turning down a challenge, driving on back roads to avoid high speeds or limited-access highways, or asking someone else to drive over the bridge. It can also be more subtle, like bringing along a friend so you are less anxious, avoiding being alone with a child to avoid unwanted thoughts, or booking only aisle seats because they give you the opportunity to quickly and unobtrusively leave if you start to feel too frightened.

Or it can be so automatic and unconscious that its avoidance function is not immediately obvious to you. It may just seem like how you cope with stress, a habit, or how you have always done things. This kind of automatic behavioral avoidance would be, for example, being too busy every evening to check a dating app, falling asleep with the television on to avoid quiet reverie, or never ever being without your cell phone. Psychologists call these kinds of actions "safety behaviors." But behavioral avoidance is just one way to keep yourself distant from these experiences.

Experiential Avoidance

Experiential avoidance involves actively focusing or refocusing your attention to keep away from some unwanted experience. This means making the effort to *not* experience the thoughts, feelings, and sensations that you are presently having. Experiential avoidance can be undertaken deliberately, or it can happen automatically and without awareness.

Sometimes experiential avoidance is simply distraction. It can be obvious, like trying to attend to something else: humming a tune or listening to a song playing in the background. Or it can be more subtle—like focusing on breathing to avoid feeling angry or changing the topic of an uncomfortable conversation. Sometimes it is in the form of shutting down, hibernating, getting bored, "vegging out," sleeping too much, not paying attention, or withdrawing. Other times, it can be providing a different drama in which to engage—like picking a fight, throwing a tantrum, or embarking on an intense conversation about something else.

Another form of experiential avoidance addresses the feeling of urgency that accompanies the alarm. If it is a false alarm, the urgency is a false urgency and should, of course, be discounted. But if there is an actual decision to be made, discounting urgency can be very problematic. The attempt to drown out any feeling of urgency is particularly evident in chronic indecisiveness, and it might look like denial, rationalization, or convenient forgetting.

If you tell yourself that there is no urgency, you can temporarily remove the stress of having to face a decision. But when this way of handling choices becomes habitual, it sets the stage for increased anticipatory anxiety and chronic indecisiveness. The stress avoidance temporarily removes the distress, functioning as a reward for putting off decisions. (We'll discuss this in more detail later in the chapter.) Experiential avoidance of urgency is often combined with behavioral avoidance, resulting in procrastination and delay, lost opportunities, and becoming stuck.

Here is a very important point: the most common and most misunderstood form of experiential avoidance is not obvious at all. It is *substituting thinking for feeling*. The direct experience of a variety of negative emotions, including anxiety, disgust, shame, sadness, uncertainty, and grief are bypassed by the active invitation of cognitive activity. This is when your thoughts might become rapid and "noisy" and function to "squeeze out" unpleasant emotions.

HELPFUL FACT—Substituting thinking for feeling is a form of avoidance.

In chapter 1, we pointed out that worry has two separate components: an initial worry thought (usually in the form of *What if [something bad happens]?*) followed by another thought that attempts to reduce the anxiety triggered by the initial thought. We pointed out that the what-if part of the worrying is anticipatory anxiety and the second half—the attempt to make the anxiety go away—often consists of rational disputation, planning, analyzing, or "coping" that actually functions as experiential avoidance. When the second part of worry keeps repeating and circling and looping, it is called "rumination."

You might engage in these repetitive ruminations, which are attempts to solve unsolvable problems or answer unanswerable questions, by substituting thinking activity for feelings. This is an attempt, often unwitting, to block the uncomfortable feelings that come with the what-if parts of uncertainty, doubts, and not knowing for sure. Rumination may seem like just part of worrying, but if you look closely at it, you will see that this second part is actually deliberate and intentional and can be changed once you understand it.

This may seem counterintuitive. It is not until we remember the two distinct parts of worrying that it becomes clear why substituting thinking for feeling backfires. Here is a simple example: *What if I ask them out and they reject me?* (Anxiety automatically goes up.) *Well, then you can always find someone else, right?* (Anxiety deliberately brought down.) Followed by, *Yes, but what if I just can't find anyone? I will always be alone.* (Anxiety automatically goes up.) Followed by, *Don't worry, someone will come along.* (Anxiety deliberately brought down.) Followed by, *You can't know that for sure.* (Anxiety automatically up again.)

This is what makes worry such a curious experience. Worry not only increases anxiety by triggering the alarm system, but it also *reduces* anxiety by increasing prefrontal cortex activity, which then cools off the system that generates your alarm reactions. When your brain is involved in thinking, planning, and analyzing—functions that engage prefrontal cortex activity—there is also a concurrent reduction of activity in the fear circuitry (Arco and Mora 2009; Wu et al. 2019). This means that the second part of worrying—the attempt to find a solution to the what-if thought—actually reduces the intensity of limbic activity (the brain circuitry that triggers the alarm response), thereby reducing the experience of anxiety. So, the rumination part of worry also functions as an avoidance.

> HELPFUL FACT—Worry both increases and decreases anxious arousal in a continuous loop.

Another form of experiential avoidance is the substitution of a different negative emotion for anxiety. This is often an automatic reaction. It is not unusual to feel the whoosh of arousal with an anxious thought or image and then immediately launch into anger or self-shaming or even sadness, entirely skipping over the anxiety.

One patient became anxious after hearing that his young daughter fell in a playground incident. His imagination instantly flashed a picture of her with serious injuries, although, in fact, she was able to quickly resume her activities. He found himself getting angry at the parent who was supervising the children. Then he started blaming himself for not sufficiently researching that parent and the safety measures at the playground. He felt duped and deceived although he also acknowledged that his reaction was wildly overblown. These feelings took him away from the direct experience of anxiety, if only for brief moments.

For those of you who are less disturbed by angry emotions than by anxiety, you may habitually feel irritated, frustrated, or angry instead of anxious. For others, the instant go-to emotion is self-critical shaming or feeling hopeless or defeated. These substitutions don't feel good, but they do accomplish the task of experiential avoidance and reinforce the tendency toward more anticipatory anxiety.

Finally, if you use habitual avoidance activities as a means of coping with your anxiety, you might have already realized that they are remarkably ineffective. In fact, all avoidance *increases* anxiety in the long run, and so your efforts are ultimately self-defeating. Understanding this basic truth about anticipatory anxiety will help point you in a direction that is far more productive.

Here are partial lists of both behavioral and experiential avoidance strategies. As you read these strategies, consider if you can identify any of them in your own life. Remember that these are just representative examples and the lists are certainly not exhaustive. And ultimately, any manner of distancing yourself from anxious feelings can be viewed as an avoidance.

Complete behavioral avoidance:

• Don't do it

- Put it off

- Don't go

- Get someone else to do it

- Get someone else to decide or choose

Partial behavioral avoidance:

- Shorten the experience

- Leave out some parts

- Avoid rush hour or crowded elevators, limit the height you are willing to go

- Go somewhere only with a companion, cell phone, or Valium

- Text to keep in contact with someone else

- Keep your escape options open

- Avoid known triggers along the way

- Listen to a podcast during the experience

- Use deliberate distraction activities

Cognitive rituals:

- Wear the *right* shirt

- Step onto the elevator with the *right* foot

- Repeat comforting phrases, such as "God is good, and God wouldn't hurt me"

- Remind yourself that you can always take a Xanax

- Repeat whenever you get anxious "This is just anxiety, I will be okay."

- Go over your pros and cons list again

Ineffective coping skills (safety behaviors):

- Imagine who can be called on to help
- Always bring water, a pet, your cell phone "just in case"
- Think about washing or arranging or fixing later
- Buy everything and plan to return almost all of it later
- Decide to decide later
- Map out safety places or people "just in case"
- Repeatedly remind yourself how unlikely a catastrophe would be

Experiential avoidance:

- Focus on your breath to avoid feeling angry
- Wear sunglasses and pretend no one can see you
- Count silently until it is over
- Take a nap until you feel ready
- Play a game on your phone for distraction
- Fantasize that you are somewhere else
- Plan your escape possibilities the whole time
- Ruminate about the what-if part of your worry thoughts
- Get angry when anxiety is triggered

Next, we will explore why avoidance, and particularly the second part of worry (rationalizing, self-reassuring, analyzing, ruminating, problem solving), does not work as a solution to anticipatory anxiety. On the surface, it seems to address your anxiety, but in reality it exacerbates it.

How Avoidance Reinforces Anticipatory Anxiety and Chronic Indecisiveness

First, we'll look at how avoidance acts as negative reinforcement, which then exacerbates anticipatory anxiety. Then we will examine how avoidance results in lost opportunities for practice, evidence, and mastery, all of which work to maintain anticipatory anxiety and chronic indecisiveness.

Negative Reinforcement

Negative reinforcement is not at all what it sounds like. It has nothing to do with and is totally different from punishment.

Psychologists use the term "reinforcement" to indicate a response to a behavior that will strengthen that behavior. Most of the time, we think of reinforcement as a reward. Your dog sits; you say, "good dog"; you pet her and give her a treat. You are training your dog to obey your command. The "good dog," petting, and treat are all rewards, or—in the lexicon of psychologists—"positive reinforcers."

Positive reinforcement is adding something positive after a behavior to make that behavior stronger. *Negative reinforcement is removing something negative after a behavior, which also makes that behavior stronger.* It is important to understand that the reduction of pain or discomfort (such as anxiety) is equivalent to an increase of pleasure.

Here are some examples of negative reinforcement. If you have a wicked headache and take an aspirin to get rid of it, you are more likely to turn to that aspirin next time you get a headache. Your pain was reduced, and that is the negative reinforcement. Taking aspirin is the behavior that is reinforced.

Here are some other examples of negative reinforcement. You are sleeping, and your alarm goes off. That sound is annoying, and so you get out of bed and turn it off. The annoying sound is removed, and the behavior of getting out of bed and turning it off is reinforced.

One additional example: You are driving, and it starts to rain. You have difficulty seeing the road through a wet windshield. So, you turn on the windshield wipers, you get a much clearer view, and driving becomes less unpleasant. The reduction of displeasure negatively reinforces the behavior of turning on the windshield wipers. Negative reinforcement—just like positive reinforcement—is a way we learn things.

Sometimes psychologists use the terms "addition reinforcement" for positive reinforcement and "removal reinforcement" for negative reinforcement. These terms make the concepts easier to remember.

Avoidance Negatively Reinforces Anticipatory Anxiety

The desire to avoid is so powerful because it can give you almost immediate relief from your anxious feelings. Unfortunately, the relief is temporary because the reduction of anxiety negatively reinforces the anticipatory anxiety that immediately preceded it. You have surely noticed that avoidance empowers your anticipatory anxiety and disempowers you.

The following figure shows how the avoidance and negative reinforcement combine to keep your anticipatory anxiety going strong.

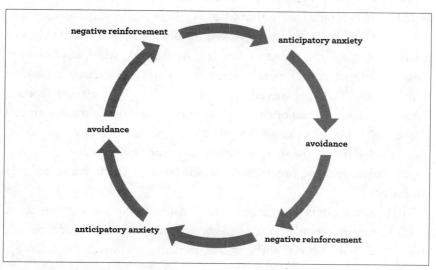

Avoidance–Negative Reinforcement Cycle

Negative reinforcement—like any reinforcement—strengthens the frequency, the intensity, and the persistence of whatever is being reinforced. This is why avoidance is so very powerful as a negative reinforcer: it makes the what-if thought more likely to return, and it increases the intensity and the persistence of the feelings that come with it.

Avoidance Blocks New Learning

Avoidance makes it impossible to check out your what-if thoughts and imagined catastrophes. It eliminates the possibility of learning that your anticipatory anxiety might be an inaccurate predictor of the upcoming event. In other words, avoidance takes away the opportunity to find out that you did not have to avoid! In fact, you tend to attribute your survival—or at least your relief—to your avoidance. ("I could not have done it without the Xanax, your support, the exit plan, or the shortened time.") And you never find out that you reacted to a paper tiger and were tricked.

When you avoid going through an experience you fear, you lose the opportunity to find out that you could handle that phone call, that you actually can ride on a bus, or that whatever you were dreading was actually not so bad. You never find out that you rapidly forget all the other choices when you just commit to one or that you are stronger, wiser, more competent, more flexible, and more able to deal with having made a mistake than you believed. You never find out that you did not need to have someone come with you or that you *can* survive an hour without your cell phone. *You never get a chance to master the experience.* You never get to see yourself adapting on the spot, learning something new, or managing to feel regret, embarrassment, or rejection and still be okay. You never get to build confidence.

In fact, without new experiences to disconfirm your assumptions about yourself, you simply rely on your memories and imagination and remain stuck. Your brain follows all the well-worn pathways. *Avoiding avoidance is how we grow.*

HELPFUL FACT—Avoidance robs you of the experience of mastery and negatively reinforces anxiety.

Self Study

If you are not moving forward—overcoming your fears and gaining confidence in your ability to make decisions in your life—there is some form of avoidance contributing to your distress. Try to identify both behavioral and experiential avoidance patterns in your own life. Some may not be immediately obvious, but knowing what is happening will make it possible to take the therapeutic steps in the rest of the book.

Conclusion

In this chapter, we delved deep into how avoidance works to keep you anxious and stuck. We explained what happens when the brain responds to triggers and creates avoidance. We described behavioral and experiential avoidance in their obvious and more subtle forms. And we have shown how avoidance works as both a negative reinforcement and a blockade against new learning.

In the next chapter, we show how anxious thinking creates distortions, hijacks your imagination, exaggerates the sense of danger, and takes over your common sense.

CHAPTER 5

Getting Hijacked by Your Imagination

For over seventeen years, I (Dr. Seif) ran the largest airport-based fear-of-flying program in the country. We met at the airport, boarded stationary planes, and—at the end of the six-week program—flew on a scheduled flight from New York to Boston. The members of this group were all terrified of flying. Some hadn't flown in ten or twenty years. Some had never flown at all. Some had made plans to travel, walked onto the plane, but then panicked and ran off just before takeoff. Most of the others had cancelled flights numerous times. Some had lost jobs because of their fear or were unable to visit loved ones who lived across the continent—or across the ocean.

Every single one of these people had a similar concern. It typically went something like this: "Once I'm on that plane, there is no turning back. If I panic, or the plane crashes, or we hit awful turbulence, I can't get out. I'm stuck in that metal tube in the sky, and that thought terrifies me so much that I just can't do it."

We came to realize that most people are terrible predictors of how they might react to a flight. Just about everyone who was brave enough to fly with the group did extremely well—not at all as they had predicted. Anticipatory anxiety produced an illusion of prediction.

In fact, every one of these fearful fliers had been misled by their imagination and fallen prey to their anticipatory anxiety. Let's take a look at why this happens.

Anxious Thinking Blocks Common Sense

You are more vulnerable to getting hijacked by your imagination if you are triggered by anxiety. It can be easy to lose track of your own good common sense. That is because anxiety changes consciousness and results in an altered state of awareness that we call "anxious thinking." Anxious thinking is the conscious consequence of your neurological alarm system reacting to an imagined danger. Since your brain is primed for danger and your autonomic nervous system is aroused, most perceptions follow a rule designed for primitive survival: assume danger until proven otherwise. And, therefore, they narrow your attention to focus vigilantly on that danger.

For that reason, anxious thinking follows a different set of rules than "regular" thinking. Your world appears different when you are coping with anticipatory anxiety and the pressure to choose when you feel unable to do so. Your altered state of awareness makes it more difficult to find—and to trust—your own good judgment. However, once you understand the ways that anxious thinking changes your perspective, it becomes much easier to find and follow it.

Here are six major reasons why it might be difficult to override your anxious thinking. These reasons also explain why you become vulnerable to believing that your own overactive imagination is serving you facts that you should attend to.

Anxious thinking selectively predicts disasters. Anxious thinking includes imagining and predicting disastrous outcomes (Seif and Winston 2014). Anxious thinking leads us to catastrophize, imagine worst-case scenarios, and focus almost exclusively on risks and much less on the possible rewards. If you consider a thousand possible outcomes when you are anxious—most of which are benign—you will spend a disproportionate amount of time and mental energy on the one or two improbable but not impossible consequences that might be disastrous. This is especially true when you are grappling with anticipatory anxiety and concerns over making a choice.

When you say to yourself that you just can't handle going to that family gathering because your ex could possibly be there and they might embarrass you, or you might panic and humiliate yourself in front of others, that is an example of catastrophizing. Another example is when you continuously cancel the MRI that your doctor says she wants to diagnose your stomach pain. Sometimes you believe that you couldn't tolerate being enclosed in the MRI and you fear that you might cancel midtest, and other times you worry that the doctor will diagnose you with a fatal illness.

The chances of your worst-case scenario coming true are small but not zero. However, the selective negativity of anxious thinking makes it seem highly likely. And, when imagining that possibility, your reaction is exaggerated by your increased state of autonomic arousal.

In nonanxious states, you recognize and accept that there are no absolute guarantees about anything and are able to proceed with the assumption that most likely things will be okay and if they are not, you will manage. Anxious minds paint vivid pictures of disasters, and you can become riveted and disabled by those images while ignoring all the other possibilities.

Anxious thinking intensifies the feeling of risk. Whenever you consider taking an action, you understand that there is some risk involved, and you implicitly weigh that risk against any possible gains. Want to take a walk around your neighborhood? You might get run over by a car or fall and break your leg. But you take your walk anyway. You have implicitly decided that the odds of something dire happening during your walk are extremely low, and so you dismiss them and take your walk. In fact, most of the time you may not even think about the risks of much of what you do each day because you have already decided that the risks are so low it makes sense to just ignore them.

When we are not anxious, how risky an action feels is a natural combination of how likely it is that the bad thing might occur (the odds of it happening) and how bad it would be if it did, indeed, occur (the stakes involved).

But anxious thinking changes that. It tends to focus only on the stakes and leaves out the odds. Let's suppose that you are about to take your walk but hear on the local news that an out-of-control car has run into a person on the sidewalk, one block from where you live. You might become frightened and think, *Oh my goodness, I could have been there! I could have been injured or killed!* In this state, your anxious thinking would make it feel dangerous to take a walk. The extremely low odds don't count, and what rivets your attention are the stakes: *What if I had been there? What if I had been run down? What if I had died on my walk?* You would feel an urge to avoid walking on the street.

Here is another example of how we might handle a weird thought differently depending on whether we're in an anxious state or not. Most people have had the experience of the sudden intrusive thought of jumping or falling off a balcony. It just passes because it is deemed as silly and unimportant. It does not feel risky to stay on the balcony. On the other hand, if a person is generally anxious about their mental health and checking to make sure they are okay, such a thought can set off an alarm and suddenly feel like a meaningful warning about risk—and there is an urge to go inside immediately.

In fact, human beings are terrible at risk assessment. The most important factor in determining how risky we view an activity is how often we engage in it! Frequent exposure reduces the feeling of risk. Even people who work in decidedly dangerous jobs report that after they have been in that job for a while, they feel safe at work. This is why "trust your gut" is not a very helpful or reliable suggestion when trying to make decisions about what is safe and what is not, what to choose and what to avoid.

> **HELPFUL FACT**—"Trust your gut" is not a very reliable suggestion about safety.

Anxious thinking emphasizes selective memory. A fifty-eight-year-old woman was terrified of public speaking. She related two experiences of intense anxiety during recent presentations and claimed that she couldn't remember a time when she was able to present without terror. After successful treatment and presenting a speech with relatively low anxiety, she suddenly remembered numerous speeches that she had given over the past forty years that were free of excessive anxiety!

This is not an uncommon phenomenon. After initially having no recall of routine problem-free functioning, people who are in recovery suddenly remember previous instances of positive interactions with others, successful completions of tasks without endless indecision, and nonanxious contact with people and situations. People struggling with intense anticipatory anxiety and indecision think of themselves as having had these problems in every instance when that is clearly not true.

We now know that memory is not a photographic record of our past. In fact, memory is elusive and retrospectively revised. Perhaps you have had the experience of discovering that a firmly held memory is actually false, distorted, or in stark disagreement with someone else's recall. Psychologists have discovered that we all remember experiences with highly charged emotions much more vividly and much more intensely than those that lack emotional intensity (Kensinger 2009). This is why anxious thinking can present you with only memories of mistakes, failures, losses, and embarrassments while minimizing past successes or emotionally neutral events, thereby persuading you that what you are facing will be as distressing as those memories.

Psychologists have also discovered the Zeigarnik effect (Koffka 1935), where people recall unfinished or interrupted tasks in far more detail than those that are finished and checked off the list. When you try to do something but avoid it or become stuck and are unable to proceed, that becomes an unfinished task. That stays in your memory, along with the anxiety and indecision that accompanied your effort. So abandoned attempts to accomplish tasks are exquisitely recalled and completed tasks are more easily forgotten.

Anxious thinking promotes the fallacy of thoughts as warnings. In an earlier book (Winston and Seif 2017), we addressed a variety of misunderstandings and myths about thought. Here are some of the myths that contribute to anticipatory anxiety and chronic indecisiveness.

Myth: Thinking something makes it likely to happen. This is a complete misunderstanding of what is known about thoughts. Psychologists call this myth "thought-action fusion" (Amir et al. 2001; Salkovskis 1985) or "magical thinking." The fact is that a thought is not a message about what is going to happen. Similarly, a thought is not a prediction or warning of an awful future action or occurrence. Thoughts do not warn of plane crashes, automobile accidents, or natural disasters. And certainly, our thoughts cannot make actions or events happen. Thoughts do not change probabilities in the real world. They do not move objects, nor can they hurt people.

Myth: Thinking something makes it unlikely to happen. This is the exact opposite of the previous myth. An example is worrying about someone as a way of protecting them or staying loyal to them. Thoughts do not change probabilities in the real world. While worrying about someone might make you feel like you are doing something to protect them, in reality you are only training your brain to reinforce a cycle of worry. It is not irresponsible or unloving to stop trying to control events with your thoughts.

Myth: Every thought is worth thinking about. Like cable TV, we have many different channels of thought going through our mind at the same time. It is impossible to think about them all, and some channels are just full of junk or irrelevant information (like the infomercial channel or the local high school announcements). Not all are worthwhile to think about. But when an intrusive thought arrives with a whoosh—no matter the content—if you believe that all thoughts are worth thinking about, then you might choose to focus on that one thought and grant it meaning and attention it does not deserve. Your attention may be hijacked by junk.

Myth: Thoughts that repeat are important. The importance or meaning of a thought has little to do with how much it repeats. Thoughts tend to repeat if they are resisted or pushed away. Any thought that you attempt to squash is more likely to keep repeating, like *Don't think about that itchy spot,* or *Stop noticing the piece of food in her teeth.* When we invest energy in any thought, it builds up neural connections and makes the thought more likely to happen (Pittman and Karle 2015). This applies to any thought, regardless of its importance. The simple fact is that attempts to keep certain thoughts from coming into your mind are what makes them come round again and feel stuck.

Anxious thinking can set up self-fulfilling prophecies. Anxious thinking views the world as hostile and threatening. If you are walking in the woods and you are told there are dangerous animals nearby, you are sure to keep to the well-worn path. Living an extremely risk-averse life means staying with the safe choice, limiting creative leaps, and eschewing novelty and the unknowns it brings. If you are too frightened to try new things, then how can you possibly succeed? We often tell our patients that—while trying something new is never a guarantee of success—the act of not trying is sure to guarantee failure. So, if you think you can't handle the situation, think you will mess up asking someone out on a date, find it too scary to drive over the bridge, or are unable to decide which shade of nail polish to purchase, you dramatically increase the chances of your fearful projections becoming reality.

There are numerous examples of this: You try to negotiate a raise for yourself but are too anxious to make a good argument for the increase. You become indecisive when someone calls for volunteers at karaoke night and miss your chance—even though you secretly practiced your song for hours. You confirm your belief that you will never become successful when you "forget" to apply for a promotion that involves worldwide travel. And you give up the chance to surprise yourself with unexpected accomplishments when you feel too frightened to try things that stretch your comfort zone.

Anxious thinking increases a feeling of urgency and reduces helpful compartmentalization. We all know about potential issues that we have no trouble setting aside until they come closer, action is required, or more information is available. But when you're anxious, whatever you are anxious about feels urgent and demanding, and you lose your ability to distract yourself from it, put it aside, or somehow "put it in a box." Once you start anxious thinking, worry marches front and center and becomes preoccupying and demanding of your attention. It pushes everything else out of the way. This is particularly true of anticipatory anxiety. And this is why "just let it go" is not advice that anxious thinking lets us follow. The worry is too sticky to let go.

Psychologists call the capacity to both know and not know something "dissociation." (It is also sometimes called "healthy repression," Wang et al. 2019.) Dissociation can serve us well; for example, it allows us to enjoy a TV show before bedtime and then fall asleep easily even when we know something big will be happening the next day. The same capacity accounts for us knowing, in the abstract, that fatal car accidents happen while still being able to comfortably drive every day. We need some helpful dissociation to be able to disentangle ourselves from worries so we can gain perspective, see the larger picture, and let time pass. Anxious thinking tends to limit our ability to access helpful (enough) dissociation.

But there is an optimum level of dissociation. If anxiety is overwhelming, the high state of distress can result in too much dissociation. This is particularly true if trauma is present, but too much dissociation can happen to anyone in a high state of painful autonomic arousal. For some people, this is what explains unconscious but convenient forgetting of important dates, appointments, and commitments during anticipatory anxiety and what makes it possible to delay and procrastinate for some people with chronic indecisiveness.

Resistance Is Futile: The Principle of Paradoxical Effort

"Paradoxical effort" refers to the idea that when it comes to anxious or unwanted thoughts and feelings, effort works backward. This is particularly relevant because anxious thinking produces a narrowed focus on danger along with an increased sense of urgency to get away. This urgency often produces an escalating urge to try even harder.

In the external world, effort produces direct results. If you want a table moved, you push or carry it to where you want it to go. There is a positive correlation between the effort you expend and the progress you make.

Work harder at digging a hole or clearing up a room, and you will have a larger hole and a cleaner room.

In the internal world, and especially when we are addressing anticipatory anxiety and chronic indecisiveness, this relationship becomes topsy-turvy. The harder you try to rid yourself of troubling thoughts or anxious feelings, the more stuck and ingrained they become. Psychologist and worry expert David Carbonell (2016) likes to say, "You are not anxious *despite* your best efforts. You are anxious *because* of your best efforts" (79). When effort is paradoxical, the best thing you can do—and often the hardest thing as well—is to do nothing and simply allow time to pass.

If sheer well-intentioned effort and willpower could overcome these problems, you would not be reading this book. You simply cannot use effort to stop thinking or to banish an unwanted thought, feeling, image, or sensation that pops up and intrudes into your awareness. Just as you cannot "unhear" the argument at the next table in the restaurant no matter how hard you try, you cannot "unfeel" the sensations of anxious arousal, such as a pounding heart or sweating palms. And, if you have an intrusive thought of something disgusting or abhorrent and engage with effort to make it go away, it sticks and returns more forcefully.

Granted, you can redirect your attention or distract yourself for a while, and you can deliberately think about something else while you are aware of the anxious thoughts and feelings. And you may very well be able to force yourself to do something (white-knuckling), but your takeaway in those cases is that you survived an ordeal, which does nothing to boost confidence or decrease future anticipatory anxiety.

In fact, these types of temporary behaviors—such as redirecting your attention and forcing yourself to white-knuckle—are actually forms of avoidance that we outlined in chapter 4, and avoidance tends to reinforce anxiety in the long run. Simply trying harder or trying to blast through your anxiety with willpower—no matter how brave and well-intentioned you may be—will not ultimately result in lasting benefits.

Anticipatory anxiety, if you let it be and leave it alone, tends to subside. If you debate it or work on it—when you ruminate or avoid it in any of the ways we presented—it intensifies. Trying hard to calm down—with frantic urgency and while demanding success—is as paradoxical as screaming at yourself to fall asleep "or else."

You already know that once you have replayed a memory of having had a panic attack on that bridge, followed your imagination into a humiliating scenario, or started monitoring your tendency to "think the worst," you are not easily able to convince yourself to ignore, refute, or argue yourself out of anticipatory anxiety. The harder you try, the stickier your thoughts get, and you are unable to reassure yourself for more than a few minutes.

Paradoxical effort can explain why many people just end up giving up and start seeing their problems as intractable or "just how they are." We strongly disagree with this conclusion and are offering you an entirely different approach to overcoming your anticipatory anxiety and chronic indecisiveness.

> HELPFUL FACT—Effort works backward when dealing with anxiety: the more effort you put into struggling with anxiety, the stronger and stickier it becomes.

A Pattern, Not a Personality Trait

Many people with a history of anticipatory anxiety or chronic indecision long ago incorporated these problems into their view of themselves. these are self-critical, judgmental beliefs about their character: "I am a procrastinator. I am unreliable. I am lazy. Don't expect me to make a commitment or meet a deadline." Others translate their anxiety and paralysis of action into low self-esteem: "I am dependent, fragile, not self-confident, needy, not brave."

A few see their behavior as justifiable or an admirable personality trait they try to defend despite the limitations on their freedom that they endure: "I am just more detail-oriented, careful, thorough, and appropriately cautious than most people." They feel justified in their avoidance and are in denial about the negative impacts of avoiding choices or reasonable risks.

And others are so used to avoiding anything that makes them anxious that they have lost their ambitions to grow, explore, experiment, or have adventures and new experiences. They sound like this: "I don't care to travel," "I am a homebody," or "I like my routines."

Defining yourself as a someone who is destined to always be a "nervous person," who doesn't enjoy doing new things, or who "is bad at" making decisions implies that you are just made this way, everyone else should accept this, and even you should not expect yourself to be any different or to learn new patterns. No matter how much you have identified your anticipatory anxiety or indecisiveness as "just who I am," you are unnecessarily limiting yourself. These ways of behaving are anxiety symptoms; they are not enduring personality traits—even if you have always been this way and even if generations in your family are similar. You are not stuck being like this if you are willing to consider other ways of relating to your inner anxious dialogues, your anxious false alarms, and your doubts.

HELPFUL FACT—Anticipatory anxiety and chronic indecisiveness are patterns, not unchangeable personality traits.

Self Study

Now that you've had the chance to consider how your anticipatory anxiety manifests and perpetuates itself, identify how your anxious thinking makes you vulnerable to being hijacked by your imagination. See if you believe some or all the myths about what thoughts mean and what they can do, and whether you are relying on your "guts" or your "feelings" in an unhelpful way.

Conclusion

This chapter explored the ways that anxious thinking hijacks your imagination, exaggerates the feeling of urgent danger, and instigates anticipatory anxiety and chronic indecisiveness. It described how thinking changes when anxiety is triggered and how you can lose track of your usual commonsense abilities to measure risk and make decisions based on facts as opposed to worries.

CHAPTER 6

Fueling Indecisiveness: Perfectionism, Desire for Certainty, and Fear of Regret

In chapter 2, we defined chronic indecisiveness as the habit of avoiding a decision—sometimes important, sometimes seemingly trivial—so you become stuck at a choice point and are unable to progress. We also noted that there is often a mutual interplay between anticipatory anxiety and chronic indecisiveness; frequently, anticipatory anxiety underlies chronic indecisiveness, and indecision often exacerbates and energizes anticipatory anxiety.

No matter the specific situation, chronic indecisiveness is intensified by three issues that we examine in this chapter: the drive toward perfection, the desire for certainty, and the fear of regret.

The Pursuit of Perfection

We define "perfectionism" as the need or intense desire to be—or to appear—flawless. Perfectionism involves setting extremely high standards for oneself and then setting out to achieve those standards. Self-evaluation is rigidly based on whether you achieve those standards. Perfectionism is based on an inflexible all-or-nothing type of thinking. If you are a perfectionist, then you are either perfect or not.

Perfectionism has no place for grey areas. Differences are not better or worse; they are either right or wrong. You view your choices and your accomplishments through the same skewed perspective: they are either flawless, or they are not. In its most extreme form, you derive no pleasure or satisfaction from your accomplishments unless your internal and external judgments rate you as perfect.

Most perfectionists are too sophisticated to believe that they could be totally flawless. After all, to err is human, and absolute perfectionism leaves no room for this human trait. So, you might tell yourself that you just want to be "as good as you possibly can be." Unfortunately, this doesn't insulate you from the desire to be as perfect as possible and the same all-or-nothing way of thinking ("your very best" or "not your very best").

You may value this way of thinking—despite the enormous demands and trouble it can bring—because it carries with it the illusion that it is the main reason why you succeed. You attribute your accomplishments to your perfectionism and therefore value it. You may have received big rewards for your achievements in terms of success, admiration, and approval and are therefore reluctant to give it up. You may think that giving up perfectionistic tendencies will make you unmotivated, sloppy, or mediocre.

However, whenever you want to be as close to perfect as you possibly can, you trap yourself in an evaluation system that focuses on flaws and mistakes. *Perfectionists don't rate themselves on how well they do; they focus on how much they fall below their desired standard.* Imagine taking a test where you get no credit for correct answers but get penalized for every wrong one. You would fret over every answer, worried that even one error would destroy your chances of passing. That is the world that perfectionists inhabit. No wonder decisions become excruciatingly difficult! Perfectionism leaves no room for mistakes. Leaving no room for mistakes leads directly to intense pressure on every choice or decision. This is an awful formula for living if your goals are learning, growing more confident in your decisions, and adding to your repertoire of skills.

We start every new experience as a beginner. Remember that the most expert, most self-assured individual you know started out as a rank beginner. Almost always, beginners feel awkward, anxious, and uncomfortable and yet proceed to make choices along with or in spite of these emotions. And, if you wait to proceed until your awkwardness or anxiety dissolves, you might wait forever! Here again, the all-or-nothing thinking of your perfectionism paralyzes you into nonaction and nonchoice.

Perfectionism preaches that mistakes can never be erased, forgotten, or compensated for. It suggests that first impressions are of lasting importance (you get "no second chances"), so you need to be "in the groove" whenever you interact with another person. It leaves no room for the idea of doing "well enough." And, if the only way to totally avoid making mistakes is to do nothing, then the habit of not making choices and being stuck is precisely what it demands. The drive for perfection is a little like hard wiring your amygdala to stay in the freeze part of the fight-flight-freeze response. Perfectionism naturally leads to paralysis.

But imagine if you weren't so demanding of yourself. What if you could believe that each mistake you make gives you the opportunity to do better the next time? What if feeling embarrassed about something was a temporary experience that led to positive change? What if you could focus on the positive aspects of imperfection, as opposed to the catastrophic ones?

Chesterton (1956), a Christian philosopher, advocated that anything worth doing is worth doing badly. His point was that the value of an activity was in the individual growth and pleasure it brings and not necessarily the goal reached or the perfect process. The challenge is to live with the paradox of learning, experimenting, and growing toward your goal of accepting "good enough" along the way.

The irony here, as we said, is that most people value the effort to be perfect because they falsely attribute their successes to it, as if giving up that unattainable ideal might start an inevitable slide to mediocracy, apathy, and failure. In fact, when hardworking, well-intentioned people abandon perfectionism, what happens is not mediocrity but excellence. And a much more joyful experience of any sort of effort. The mean task-master of perfectionism makes necessary uncertainties intolerable, takes the pleasure out of learning, and paralyzes you in the face of choices and decisions.

Your perfectionism is likely anchored in values about effort, responsibility, and ethics. You do not need to abandon these values but rather consider the consequences of the rigid and unforgiving application of them. Inflexibility leaves you overemphasizing some activities to the detriment of others. If aiming for perfection at work takes you away from family, or if devoting too many hours to achieving error-free emails robs you of needed sleep, you lose other valued sources of satisfaction.

Perfectionism is also the enemy of creativity. When you become overly concerned about doing things just right, you become risk averse and find it increasingly difficult to take the leap of faith that corresponds to every significant creative effort. Steve Jobs, the founder of Apple, Inc., was a remarkably creative person whose willingness to take risks allowed personal computing to make quantum leaps. And, even though plenty of his decisions turned out to be unproductive, Jobs never stopped making creative choices while accepting the possibility that they might be wrong. In fact, he left Apple to create a totally different company, one that never succeeded as a business venture, before returning to Apple over ten years later. This part of his career is not what we remember.

Perfectionism is the breeding ground of unrealistic expectations. If you expect yourself to be close to flawless, you will always be disappointing yourself. Making the right choice is burdened with the task of protecting your self-esteem and self-worth. If your decisions can only be great or awful, then you tend to value yourself in the same all-or-nothing category. So, you invariably lose self-confidence and put even more pressure on yourself to be perfect next time. Perfectionism leaves no room for self-compassion or for valuing who you are rather than what you accomplish.

Some perfectionists believe that it protects them in the eyes of others—that they would lose respect without it or that mistakes would have dire consequences for how they would be perceived. But the reality is that most people don't really notice or care. They are often too busy paying attention to themselves. And your idea of being perfect is probably quite different from others. When working with people who are focused on making perfect public speeches, Carl Robbins (2016) asks them to stop in the middle of the presentation and pause for ten or fifteen seconds—deliberately "ruining" their flawless speech. Most listeners don't even notice the pause, and those who do assume that it is a lead-up to some important point. It grabs their attention and makes the speech more interesting.

There are many studies indicating that perfectionistic people tend to be judged by others as more critical, more hostile, and less likeable than those who are seen as nonperfectionistic (Hewitt et al. 2019; Davis et al.

2018). This is the exact opposite of the (false) belief that mistakes lower your respect and likability. Striving for a perfect speech may result in avoiding setting the date, revising the draft endlessly, and never feeling ready to commit to the speech. So, striving for a perfect speech is both impossible and ill-advised.

Since perfectionism is intrinsically linked to all-or-nothing thinking, it is a common partner to catastrophic thinking. Choices are seen as right or wrong, so outcomes then become either good or bad. Every decision becomes incredibly important since one wrong choice can lead to the complete collapse of the series of "just right" outcomes required to achieve that perfect result. One multiple-choice question mistake on a high school quiz can be the fly in the ointment that spoils one's chances of getting into an elite college, finding a great job, meeting a life partner, and having a life worth living. Similarly, buying a house that is not guaranteed to increase sufficiently in value could destroy one's entire financial plan. One patient believed that they would not be able to stand it if they disappointed a friend, which led them to avoid having friends, as the burden they placed on themself to be a perfect friend was too great. Catastrophic thinking driven by perfectionism elevates every choice to a potential disaster, fueling both anticipatory anxiety and the reluctance to commit to any choice.

In extreme cases, small decisions that ought to be simple become agonizing and feel like dangerous risks. One patient, while debating whether or not to train her dog with an invisible fence, imagined that the wrong choice could lead to the dog being run over, her daughter blaming her for the death, and the need to commit suicide to atone for her mistake. Another patient kept changing his mind about which shoes to buy because every option was too expensive or too cheap or too fashionable or not fashionable enough, resulting in no new shoes at all. His intolerable risk was the imagined story that he would wear the shoes once, then not like them, and it would be too late to send them back—and he would feel so bad about having wasted money that he would lose his girlfriend because of being no fun to be with, and he would never find true love.

> HELPFUL FACT—Perfectionism paralyzes by leaving no room for any mistakes.

The Desire for Certainty

When you think about it, there is very little in life that we can be certain of. Uncertainty is inherent in every decision we make, from the most profound choices of our lives (*Have I chosen the right person as my partner? If I take this job, will it advance my career?*) to the most mundane (*What color should I paint my room? Is this purchase a good deal? What should I have for breakfast?*). We can have doubts about virtually anything (*Am I really a good person? Will this plane crash? Could I have an asymptomatic illness?*). Most of the time we are confident enough in our choices—or that they just don't matter that much—that we can bypass our doubts enough to make plans and follow through with some assurance.

However, for those with chronic indecisiveness, the uncertainties and doubts that each potential choice unleashes become barriers that stop the decision process in its tracks. In fact, studies have shown that the need to know for sure—the problem many have with tolerating uncertainty—is a major reason why so many suffer from anxiety (Grupe and Nitschke 2013). It is the paramount contributor to chronic indecisiveness. The need to know for sure can immobilize you. Let's take a look at what it actually means when we say that we are sure of a choice.

The Question of Certainty

Every assumption you make about the world is imbued with uncertainty, from the most trivial (my pen has ink) to the most profound (my parent, partner, child is alive). In fact, you can't be sure of either until you check. (And then right after you check, you can no longer be certain because things can change.) Still, most people feel certain enough, and that is sufficient to keep them comfortable even without checking. But if you experience chronic indecisiveness, the desire to be certain is spoiled by feeling so much doubt. So, let us now take a closer look at the experience of doubting.

The experience of uncertainty is different from not having enough facts. It is a kind of thought called a "metacognition" accompanied by a feeling. We explore metacognition in the next chapter, but for our purposes here, uncertainty is the awareness or knowledge that we do not know something for sure. The awareness is most often accompanied by a feeling about not knowing. The feeling can be excitement (*Who is going to win this football game?*) or fear (*What if I cannot handle what happens?*) or shame (*If that were to happen, I would never be able to live with myself.*) or any other feeling. Occasionally, uncertainty is just neutral (*I don't know for sure whether I said that, but I don't really care.*).

> HELPFUL FACT—Anxious uncertainty is an uncomfortable awareness of not knowing something for sure.

Some ordinary doubts can simply be resolved enough with facts. (*Is that the right name of this movie star? Did I finish my sandwich or leave it on my plate earlier? Did I forget to send that email I was thinking about?*) This kind of doubt can be settled by using your senses to look and see what is currently true. (*Yes, that is his name. Yes, there is nothing left on my plate. Yes, I did forget; that email was not sent.*)

However, there is a different kind of doubt that arises from your imagination—and no amount of fact-checking will ever resolve the doubt and allow you to feel certain enough. Your imagination can make you doubt what you have perceived from your senses. Here is an example. A doubt arises: *Did I turn the stove off?* You check, and your senses tell you yes. You feel sure. But then, as you walk away, another kind of doubt arises that is an imagined narrative of what you just saw. *What if I checked too hastily, or what if I turned it back on when I checked it, or what if it did not turn it off completely, or what if I burn down the house, and what harm would it do to check again?* This kind of doubting cannot be settled with another "fact" because it is generated by your imagination: you can always come up with another story with a bad outcome. No matter how many times you attempt to settle it with a reassurance or a check, you are never able to feel sure enough.

Other examples of doubting arise from your imagination about the future. Here again, facts are of no help in allowing you to feel sure enough. It might be a worry that something from the past will return with bad consequences, or you realize that you have no guarantees about the outcome of a choice in the future. *(Will I have a panic attack if I go? Have I inadvertently made a bad decision I do not even know about? How can I be sure I will remain healthy?)*

Being aware of an unwelcome possibility—and being unable to recognize clearly that you have inadvertently made up a story that scares you—makes it difficult to ignore. No matter how slim the probability that the bad outcome could happen, it is a real possibility—and now that you have imagined it, it seems to urge you to do something: be responsible, prevent a bad thing from happening, resolve this doubt, find a way to avoid something. The problem, of course, is that there are no facts in the concrete here and now that can help you resolve this. *The story resides in your imagination.* And this kind of obsessional doubt actually increases the more you engage with it, either by thinking about it more and more or by checking for new facts. You have already dismissed your common sense in favor of a preoccupation with your unresolvable doubts.

Choices therefore create a hugely difficult issue if you are chronically indecisive. Each choice you make starts you on a different path. Sometimes it is trivial *(If I choose a red purse, then my whole outfit needs to match)*; sometimes it could be consequential *(If I buy this house, I am committing to a long commute)* or even life altering *(If I accept this job, I am committing to this career path)*. So, can you ever be certain that you are making the right choice? When you acknowledge the reality that unexpected things happen and unexpected consequences are likely to show up from time to time, you realize that you can never really know for sure. All you can do is *feel* sure. Even so, many people can put their uncertainty in the background and feel *sure enough* to carry on. Knowing for sure is not about nailing down certainty, banishing doubts, or gathering more facts. It is not about telling yourself that you can be certain, that all will be well, that there is no reason to have any doubts. It is really about feeling sure enough.

People with chronic indecisiveness often find that just making a choice becomes torturous because feeling sure enough is elusive. You become overwhelmed with concerns *(Am I making an irrevocable mistake? Am I embarking on a path I can't handle? Will this lead to a wasted life? What if my choice is wrong?)* that trigger anxiety, so delay, avoidance, and procrastination seem to be the only acceptable options. And, for many, the same paralysis stemming from not feeling sure enough can engulf them when making even the most trivial of decisions: *Which exit should I take from the parking lot? Should I get a double latte or just a regular hot coffee?* In situations like these, you might even ask yourself, *Why do I have such difficulty making up my mind when it really doesn't matter?* When you are stuck this way at a trivial choice point, it is the anxiety caused by your uncertainty that you are avoiding, rather than any negative consequences of making a mistake. So you genuinely become incapable of viewing your alternatives with any degree of objectivity or common sense.

> HELPFUL FACT—When you can't make a small decision, you are avoiding the feeling of uncertainty, not the specific consequences of your choice.

Some may take the tactic of waiting for the right time to make a choice. How many times have you said to yourself something similar to this: *I'm looking for a rug for my bedroom, but there might be great sales next week, or next month, or next President's Day?* You wait and delay and—guess what?—you've been without a bedroom rug for years and are still no closer to finding one at the right price. The problem is that you just can't know for sure when is the best time to buy the right rug. There is no getting around uncertainty.

You may be a dedicated researcher, devoting time and energy to finding the right place to live, the most reliable car, or the most well-suited primary-care physician. Or you may date one person after another, diligently looking for "the one." But every answer you get leads to another set of questions, and you somehow never end up with enough information to find the place to live, purchase the car, choose the doctor, or make a commitment. Here again, the real culprit is that you just can't know for sure, and your efforts don't address your difficulty in tolerating the uncertainty that accompanies every decision.

In the effort to bypass the discomfort of uncertainty, you maintain the hope that somehow—in some inexplicable manner—the right choice will just speak to you and communicate in an unwavering and undeniable manner that says, "HERE I AM. CHOOSE ME. I'M THE RIGHT

CHOICE." Unfortunately, you will be waiting for a very long time to hear that voice, and probably it will never come.

When overwhelmed with the burden of making a decision, it is not uncommon for your mind to go blank and to feel enervated to the point of exhaustion. So you wait, hoping for inspiration that will provide the motivation and confidence in yourself you need to once again carry on. The problem here is that you are reversing the order by which both motivation and confidence are developed. In real life, *action precedes both confidence and motivation:* the first steps make it easier to take additional ones. Your brain is wired to become more comfortable with, more confident in, and more motivated to proceed with actions that you perform more frequently. IBM—the computer company—recognized this truism when it changed its corporate motto from "Think" to "Action."

The Key Shift

Your attempts to fix your apprehension about not knowing for sure are most probably leading you in the wrong direction. Waiting for the right time, hoping for inspiration and motivation, overdoing your research—these are all attempts to eliminate uncertainty from your decision making. A much more productive approach is to work toward feeling more comfortable with your discomfort. That approach tackles head-on the impossibility of eliminating uncertainty and helps you train your brain and body to function well amid uncertainty. The goal is to help you feel sure enough of your decisions to carry on with self-confidence. We will address this in much more detail starting in chapter 7 when we introduce the therapeutic attitude and metacognitive perspective.

The Fear of Regret

The fear of regret is anxiety about doing something you might later regret. It intensifies the inaction and paralysis of chronic indecision, a direct consequence not only of having a rich imagination for all the scenarios that could go wrong, but also a belief that should there be a mistake or a negative consequence, or should you be responsible for having made a wrong choice or done something too risky, your regrets would be unbearable. You can look ahead and think that you might be making a terrible mistake by putting your savings in a particular investment or purchasing a particular used car. Or you end up not being able to make a phone call because you imagine how you might feel if it becomes awkward and then you regret having made the call. You automatically imagine the awful consequences of everything going wrong and may feel that you could not stand it or could not go on. It can be especially paralyzing if you believe you are not well equipped to handle regret. You may imagine that you will never be able to get over it and will suffer endlessly. With those kinds of stakes in mind, it is no wonder that moving forward becomes problematic.

Regret occurs in a variety of situations. You are experiencing regret when you look back at a choice point and say to yourself, *Why didn't I know?* or *How could I have done something like that?* or most commonly, *IF ONLY I had not done that.* Regret can also come about if you have made a choice in the past that failed to fulfill some moral or practical obligation or started a chain of events resulting in harm to yourself or others. You can also feel regret when you have done something that has not caused any real trouble but has stimulated doubts, worries, or some other emotional distress because it seems in retrospect to have been "too risky," impulsive, or ill-considered. In the same vein, regret can happen if you did not take an action that you now wish you had.

Anticipation of regret can also happen if you are ambivalent about two possible choices. Ambivalence occurs when both choices seem either equally attractive or equally distressing, and choosing one means not choosing the other, leaving it behind. In cases where neither choice seems good, *The grass might be greener if I choose the other* can be a paralyzing thought. Even in low-stakes situations—the burger or the pasta, this hotel or that hotel, this tie or that tie?—if you believe that you might truly regret the loss of the choice left behind, you can be frozen in place, oscillating between choices. This can happen if you are anxious about being able to get past feelings in general, and it is common in people with sticky minds and anxiety sensitivity.

Regret plays some role in all our lives. We all make mistakes, and everyone can look at something they did in the past or an action they didn't do but wish they had done and wish that it were different. These can be actions that lead to regret, like losing one's temper, an infidelity, a bad investment, or even a choice of spouse. Additionally, there can be regret for what we didn't do, such as regretting turning down or not applying for a job or regretting not committing to a romantic partner. Because the costs of inaction are so often overlooked when one is paralyzed by chronic indecisiveness, regret almost always includes *I wish I had taken more chances, I regret never asking that person out,* or *I regret not having bought that birthday present for my daughter.*

Your imagination can torment you with what-ifs about experiencing humiliation, losses, failures, or any other consequence that might give you unresolvable regrets. These can branch out in all directions so it appears to be a dangerous slippery slope to do anything at all. This tendency to fear regret can be amplified if there really was something you did in the past (like most people) that was, in retrospect, a poor decision. Ruminating about a past mistake, error of judgment, or impulsive action that did in fact turn out badly is common in people with sticky minds and demanding standards.

In life, every decision we make reduces the alternatives that are available to us. If you rent an apartment, you are committed to that lease, to commuting from that area, and to sending your children to a particular set of schools. Depending on the richness of your imagination, even the most common, everyday decisions can become infused with the fear of regret: *Will I regret buying steel-cut oats instead of rolled?* or *Will I regret spending time watching a comedy on TV rather than an educational documentary?*

Because you experience instant doubts the moment you decide something—even if nothing has yet gone wrong—you approach decisions with trepidation: you understand you will have to override doubts and could regret any irreversible or final decision. Since you want to avoid the what-if uncertainty that happens automatically, you avoid the decision itself. This is the reason that commitment *without wavering* is such an important component of decision making, as well as dealing with all forms of anticipatory anxiety. It is a way of walking past the doubts that arise automatically once a decision is reached.

If you are a person with chronic indecisiveness, here is a suggestion: because instant doubts happen automatically, expect them to occur as soon as you make a decision—because they will. And if you fight them, they can throw you off guard and back to wavering. So allow them, welcome them. Be ready with the resolve that you will not explore or debate your doubts. *Just count them.* Literally. Assign each doubt a number and see how high a number you can get to. Make it a challenge to notice even subtle variations of these doubts. And see how many automatic doubts your anxious imagination comes up with in the first moments after you have made a choice. And then again, the next day. Celebrate your creativity and your astonishing ability to "yes, but" yourself, *but do not waver.* This creativity serves you well in other arenas but not in this way. We will elaborate on this shift in attitude and perspective in the next chapter.

HELPFUL FACT—Dealing with the fear of regret requires walking past doubts that arise automatically.

The fear of regret is often a component of the FOMO patterns discussed in chapter 2. The reluctance to close any pathways, opportunities, or options is fueled by the anticipation of wishing retrospectively that you had not limited yourself by making a choice. It is very common in people with high anxiety sensitivity because there is now an additional worry: not only the fear that regret may happen but also the belief that you could not stand it, that you would never get over it, or that the experience of regret would be catastrophic.

The fear of regret can prevent you from moving forward. But it can also be an obstacle to enjoying the path you have already taken. As soon as a choice is made, doubts arise, and you feel uncertain about the future possible bad outcomes or consequences. The satisfaction of a choice well made or a job well done becomes elusive because you are always worried that a decision you made in the past will lead you to regret it sometime in the future.

HELPFUL FACT—The worry that "what if" could turn into "if only" can stop you from moving forward.

Staying undecided is a way of protecting yourself from potential imagined regrets, which is how fear of regret fuels chronic indecisiveness. Ironically, in the desperate effort to avoid the pain of endless deliberations and doubts without getting anything accomplished, sometimes a rash or impulsive decision is made, often with less-than-desirable consequences. One patient said, "I've been sitting on the fence for such a long time I can't stand it. I no longer care which choice I make. I just want to get off." The desire to reduce the discomfort of uncertainty can override the obsessive decision-making process and set you up to make reckless choices.

Bypassing Perfectionism, Uncertainty, and Fear of Regret

Fortunately, although you may not realize it, you have at your disposal what everyone has: your best guess based on your own good common sense. One way of getting in touch with that is the gun test, a mental experiment described by the OCD expert Jonathan Grayson (2014). Here is one adaptation of what he calls the gun test:

> Let's suppose that you are faced with a choice and feel indecisive. Imagine that I know which is the best choice, and I have a gun to your head. I say to you, "I know the right choice, and I want you to make that decision right now. If you make the wrong choice, I pull the trigger. If you delay more than ten seconds, I pull the trigger. In both cases, you are dead. Now, make your best guess in order to save your life. Go!"

In this situation, with the stakes at the maximum, you have almost no time to think or to imagine the various untoward consequences. Instead, you have to take action and just make a choice. You aren't certain, but the (pretend) certainty of having a gun at your head takes precedence, and you take your best guess to save your life. This is the value of the gun test. It identifies your best guess as the only option you really have and allows you to abandon the impossibility of knowing for sure.

HELPFUL FACT—After learning the facts, your best guess is really the only option you ever have.

After making a choice based on the gun test, you will find that you can acknowledge that you were pretty sure about your choice, but just not totally certain. It was your desire for certainty, your perfectionism, and your fear of regret that were putting on the brakes. You may even acknowledge that you were 99 percent sure which way to go but couldn't take the tiny chance of being wrong, making an imperfect choice, or regretting your decision in the future.

If used properly, this kind of mental exercise is a helpful way to access your own sense of being "sure enough," "good enough," and less likely to feel regret. It clarifies for you that your primary avoidance has little to do with any external issues. Rather, you are trying to run away from doubt, imperfection, and regret.

Another illuminating exercise also helps to bypass the hesitations and paralysis of chronic indecisiveness. We call this the "coin toss." Find a coin and assign two competing choices to heads and tails. Toss the coin and then do not look at the result. Ask, instead, "Right now, am I hoping for heads or tails?" Here again, you are accessing your best guess.

Once a doubt has entered by means of your imagination (whether it is about possible imperfection, regret, or other unwanted outcomes), it cannot be undone. It is not resolvable—you will never be entirely certain—but you can carry on as if the risks are reasonable, and you can be aware that your rich imagination has pointed out possibilities that do not have to be addressed. Seeking more reassurance or facts will never result in a resolution because that is not where the doubts arise. Giving up on feeling absolutely certain is the only option.

Self Study

Did you identify how your own relationship to uncertainty, fear of regret, and perfectionism may affect your decision making?

Conclusion

Now that we have explored types of anticipatory anxiety and chronic indecisiveness, how they happen, and what factors contribute to their intensity and maintenance, we turn to a systematic look at how to change your patterns, overcome avoidance, and move forward.

CHAPTER 7

The Therapeutic Attitude: A Metacognitive Perspective

This chapter introduces what you will need in order to change the way you deal with both anticipatory anxiety and chronic indecisiveness. It involves changing your point of view by observing your experiences from a metacognitive perspective and then embracing what we call the "therapeutic attitude." In this approach, you will learn to take a step back and adopt a view of your mind and body that is broader. You will then be asked to make the attitudinal shift that changes how you relate to your anticipatory anxiety—away from viewing it as a series of approaching emergencies that need to be avoided and toward the most direct approach for recovery. The goal is to stop providing the fuel that maintains your anxiety and your intolerance of the uncertainties that are blocking action and decision making. This approach is more focused on *how* your thoughts, feelings, and sensations work to keep you suffering and stuck (the process) and less on what they are about (the content). To be able to observe what is happening as your anxious process unfolds is a prerequisite for change.

This might seem like a daunting task, but we ask that you ride out the anxiety bumps that will inevitably arise as you learn this new approach. You are likely already frustrated with your unsuccessful attempts to get rid of anticipatory anxiety. We are not talking here about specific anxiety management techniques, nor coping mechanisms—most often those techniques are forms of avoidance that don't get to the heart of the issue. Instead, we are asking you to learn a new perspective, one that steps outside of your usual way of experiencing your mind and body, paying attention to your thoughts, memories, worries, bodily sensations, expectations, emotions, and, most particularly, your *imagination*. This is actually a more profound approach, and we believe it will be worth the effort.

The Metacognitive Perspective

This perspective, called "metacognitive," is essentially the awareness of your own cognition. "Metacognition" is sometimes defined as "thinking about thinking," but we are expanding it to include being "aware of one's awareness." It also encompasses your beliefs about the contents of your mind, your evaluation of the experiences of your mind, and your relationship to those thoughts, memories, sensations, and feelings. It involves widening your perspective, taking a step back, and observing yourself. It is being able to identify the "I" in "I am thinking thoughts" as separate from the thoughts themselves.

In earlier books, we referred to a metacognitive process we call "disentanglement": the conscious act of "not getting involved" while still being aware of and not denying or pushing away what you are thinking and feeling. This means that once we stand back and watch carefully, we can see that thoughts are just thoughts, feelings are just feelings, and neither are facts. We can see that we are scaring, shaming, or frightening ourselves with our what-ifs. Disentangling from content is akin to a concept called "defusion" (Harris 2019) in which oneself and one's thoughts and feelings are separated.

> HELPFUL FACT—A metacognitive perspective disentangles you from the content of your thoughts and feelings.

You might notice the similarities between a metacognitive perspective and mindfulness. In fact, being mindful is a metacognitive stance that includes being nonjudgmental. The term "mindfulness" is now used so widely that we need to define what we mean by it. We are not talking about meditating to clear your mind, utilizing mindfulness as a relaxation technique, or "mindfully" trying to think through an issue. We are talking about observing whatever is happening, making no judgments, and then just leaving it alone.

Without this new perspective that emphasizes process instead of content, each instance of worried anticipation, each decision about avoidance, and each issue or obstacle are dealt with as separate problems. As a result, your days can be caught up in trying to solve one problem after another. Each issue seems separate and unconnected, so when you have successfully avoided one anxiety-producing event, another pops up. Like Whack-a-Mole in an amusement park, there is always another, which contributes to a general experience of life as a series of dreaded choice points, unwelcome challenges, and missed opportunities for novelty, challenge, and growth.

On the other hand, a metacognitive perspective allows you to understand that each worried anticipation, each avoidance urge, and each crisis of decision is a repetition of a common process—one that perpetuates itself and keeps anxiety going. As you observe yourself engaging in these maladaptive tactics, you create the opportunity to strengthen your ability to interrupt and make changes. This increases your confidence to reach for the things you desire, cope more comfortably with uncertainty, and make choices free from the paralysis of indecision. This is, in many ways, a much more profound change than just trying to cope with each problem as it comes along. *It is a change in the habitual process that creates your problems.*

The metacognitive perspective allows you to *attend to* the unproductive processes we outlined in earlier chapters and to shift from your typical reactions to new ones. It allows you to *observe* when you have left common sense and have been hijacked by your imagination; it allows you to *notice* when you have mistaken the automatic whoosh of a triggered false-alarm response for real danger; it allows you to *recognize* a familiar pattern of empty reassurance-seeking or excessive "research" and get it labeled as fuel for more anxiety or paralysis. It allows you to *note* subtle avoidance and perfectionistic behavior and attempt to find certainty where none can exist. It allows you to *let go of* mistaken beliefs and assumptions about your mind and your body that fuel your anxiety. It is a step back from yourself.

HELPFUL FACT—The metacognitive approach is not anxiety management nor a coping skill: it is a shift of perspective.

When you take this perspective, you can see for yourself that much of your anxiety comes not from the first whoosh of anxious arousal, but rather from your attempt to run away from it and fight it off. We explained in chapter 5 the concept of paradoxical effort: that effort works backward and resistance is futile when dealing with anxiety. Each time you fight the feeling of anxiety, the feeling of anxiety fights back harder.

The metacognitive perspective also allows you to focus on the process so the importance of the specific content of your worried thoughts recedes. This disentangling from content enables you to see something critical to your recovery. What you are struggling against is not the content of your thoughts or imaginings: you are struggling against feelings that arise from committing to choices in the face of unavoidable uncertainty. You are grappling with the possibility that you will feel incompetent to handle what might happen or regret a mistake or an outcome that is less than ideal.

You will also be able to see that your anticipatory anxiety is based on your imagination about the future—about something that has not yet happened. Your fearful feelings are not really about that event but rather about your fear of the anxiety itself and your own beliefs about what you can handle. You will be able to see that you are not really afraid of bridges, small talk, or mice, but you are afraid that your imagined story about what could happen will come true and you will not be able to handle it.

You may begin to notice that certain types of triggers automatically put you into avoidance mode. You will find that certain thoughts—what-if thoughts are prime culprits—are particularly good at hijacking your imagination and taking you across the bridge from ordinary common sense into the world of anxious thinking (O'Connor et al. 2005).

Challenging False Metacognitive Beliefs

Metacognitive beliefs are beliefs about thoughts. You might not be conscious of these beliefs, but they govern how you relate to your thoughts, how much power you give them, and how willing you might be to let thoughts pass by or allow their presence when they show up. Many of these beliefs are false and contribute to the power of your imagination to push you around.

Anticipatory anxiety rests on typical what-if worry thoughts, and there are many very common false beliefs about worry thoughts that need to be corrected. Let's look at them one at a time.

False belief: Worry means I care. One of the authors was speaking with a patient about uncertainty and used the following example: "My daughter is traveling, and I am actually not sure whether she is in the air or not right now—in fact, her travels are so complicated that I am not sure what country she is in." The patient was dumbstruck and disapproving: "Don't you care about your daughter? How can you stand not worrying about her? I need my kids to text me whenever they go anywhere, when they are leaving, and when they arrive. If I stopped worrying, doesn't that mean I have stopped caring about their safety?"

Here is the response: "Of course I care. I am just willing to accept not knowing for sure. It is not as if my worrying helps anyone. I am assuming that I would hear if there were a problem. And, I suspect that your worrying might annoy your kids because they have to stop and allay your worries as you request."

It is common for people to think that if you love someone, you must worry about their health, safety, and well-being. And that, conversely, if you do not stay "connected" to them through anticipatory anxiety and worry, then you are being careless, disloyal, undedicated, or uncaring. This is not true. It is a false metacognitive belief.

False belief: Worry prevents mistakes. A mother prided herself on being attentive to the needs of her three teenage daughters. She constantly worried about the myriad of dangers that can befall teens. She often anticipated stresses they might encounter and tried to protect them. She believed that her worrying prevented her from making parenting mistakes by keeping her focused and on the lookout. Relaxing her vigilance was not an option. The mother was horrified when one daughter admitted that she had been bullied in school but had kept it to herself. She told her mother, "You are always stepping in, and I was afraid you would make it worse." Worrying cannot prevent all mistakes and can sometimes work backward.

An insurance salesman who believed that worrying was essential to give his clients the very best service spent many sleepless nights mentally reviewing every form he filled out and every phone call he made to reassure himself that he had made no errors that could upset either his supervisor or his clients. As a result, he was sleepy and overcaffeinated each morning, which made it more difficult to concentrate. He was mortified when a supervisor pointed out that he had omitted a client's name on a form he submitted the previous morning. Here, worrying not only did not prevent mistakes, but it may have even made them more likely.

False belief: Worry can banish doubts. A young man was trying to figure out if he should ask out a coworker with whom he had had many enjoyable conversations. He was afraid of being rejected and was aware of doubts about their feelings for him. He imagined asking them out, being rejected in horror, and then being unable to remain at his job because of unbearable humiliation. He worried that the risk was just too high. He spent time every night before sleep ruminating and worrying, rerunning every interaction of the day in his mind, recalling the expression on their face, the tone of voice, and body language, trying to establish a feeling of certainty. He believed that *If I just think through this completely, I will get myself certain and will take action.* In truth, he was just replaying the same script over and over again, getting no closer to certainty, an impossibility.

False belief: Worry helps solve problems. There is a common confusion about the difference between planning and worrying. Let's clarify the distinction: Planning involves thinking about and coming up with a potential solution to a problem or a set of problems. It often starts with a what-if, and it results in an action plan that stops the thinking—at least until you find out if the plan solves the problem. If the problem is solved when the action is taken, nothing more is needed. If the problem remains, there is more thinking to provide a plan-B action plan. Here's a simple example: The low-fuel indicator on my car goes on. I "solve" this problem by detouring to the gas station. But that one is closed, so I make a plan B to drive to another one. I fill my car with gas, and the problem is solved. The key point here is that planning is productive: it has a viable action plan that you commit to taking.

Worrying often starts out just like planning, with a what-if. However, it does not result in a viable action plan. It just goes round and round in ruminating internal dialogues. This is because the worrying is an attempt to solve an unsolvable problem, answer an unanswerable question, become certain about something, or make a reasonable plan of action without enough information. Most often, the worrying is about some imagined future event with insufficient and unknowable facts. Other times, worry focuses on a real past event and the imagined terrible consequences that could occur as a result.

Unproductive worrying does not solve problems: it causes misery. Here's an example: I am concerned that it might snow next December when a friend is getting married. I am afraid to drive in the snow. What if I can't get there? What if no one is nearby to come and get me? What if I disappoint my friend? Should I tell her now that I might not go because of snow? Would that conversation make her upset with me? Should I buy a four-wheel-drive car now? Unproductive worry goes on and on...

False belief: Worry protects me. This can be viewed in two different ways: worry protects me by getting me "ready" in case something bad happens, and worry protects me from bad things happening—which can also be called "magical thinking."

You may believe that worrying provides a kind of preparatory emotional support, as if sudden bad news would be harder to handle than something you have already worried about. One patient valued her worrying about her mother's eventual death because she believed it would help her survive it if she practiced her grief ahead of time. When her mother eventually died, she realized that her anticipatory imaginings were not how she felt, and there had been a lot of pain that had served no purpose. It is a myth that dealing with something you have worried about is somehow made easier by having worried.

The illusion that worrying is protective is created by the fact that most of the catastrophes that are worried about do not come to pass. (The really bad things that befall us in life—accidents, disastrous illness, financial disaster—almost always come out of left field.) Despite all the obvious evidence to the contrary, many people maintain a belief that the act of worrying results in protection from bad things happening and even helps to bring on good ones.

Here are some common examples. Anxious fliers often believe that they should stay awake, look outside the plane, watch the flight attendants for unusual behavior, and evaluate the flight continuously—as if this will help keep the plane in the air. Somehow it feels too risky to fall asleep or read a book. Other examples include continuously "checking in" with friends to make sure they still want you as a friend ("Are we okay?"); superstitious behavior, like making sure to wear your lucky shirt to an anxiety-producing event; worrying diligently about your four-year-old getting into college; and checking your memory daily in case you might miss early signs of dementia.

False belief: The law of attraction. There is a belief that is prevalent in some new age philosophies that similar things are attracted to each other (Scott 2020). It is said that people tend to attract people who are similar and that people's thoughts attract similar consequences. This suggests that positive thoughts attract desirable experiences and negative thoughts attract bad experiences. Many also believe that "nature abhors a vacuum," so you should remove negative thoughts and "toxic" people from your life so there is room for positive ones. This is the false belief that banishing negative thoughts or negative energy is a way to control what happens in the real world, so worry thoughts are perceived as dangerous in and of themselves and must be avoided.

This is also magical thinking, bolstered by selective memory, a leap of faith, and a desire to be and do good. Unfortunately, if you are prone to anticipatory anxiety, this belief system is impossible to comply with, guilt-inducing when something bad happens, and it can be infuriating as a message from others. Urgently banishing negative thoughts makes them bounce back stronger.

False belief: Worries that pop up are warnings. Sudden intrusions of what-if thoughts arrive with a whoosh of alarm, as we reviewed in chapter 3. This makes them seem important, relevant, and requiring of attention. Our brains are primed to respond as if there is danger even when there is none. Anticipatory anxiety encourages us to treat these pop-up thoughts as warnings, signals, or, somehow, peeks into the future, as if our worries are predictions. But nothing could be further from the truth. *Worries have their origin in our imaginations, not in knowing anything about what lies ahead.* Anticipatory anxiety tells us nothing about what will happen.

One woman told me that she suddenly had the thought that her food pantry could have been exposed to a coronavirus months ago when she had shopped before the pandemic shutdown. This thought was so disturbing and compelling that she was unable to rest until she threw everything out and restocked her pantry. Another man told me that he associates "bad thoughts" with whatever he is touching at the moment. When he suddenly had the thought that his elderly mother might die while he was putting on a sock, the sock felt contaminated and like a "jinx." He felt warned—and was compelled to go check on her to make sure she was okay and to throw out the socks.

HELPFUL FACT—Worries have their origin in our imaginations, not in knowing anything about what lies ahead.

The Therapeutic Attitude Shift

The therapeutic attitude shift is a profoundly important component of recovery. It is a change in attitude—a change in your relationship with your anxiety. This attitudinal shift favors expecting, accepting, and allowing anxious feelings. It means changing the way you react to your anxious thoughts, feelings, memories, and sensations. We are asking you to make a fundamental shift in the relationship you have with your internal experience. You are working toward accessing the "you" who can observe your thoughts and feelings in a compassionate, nonjudgmental manner—a "you" who can neither be bullied, overwhelmed, nor shamed by whatever your imagination has come up with or by whatever sensations your automatic fight-flight-freeze reaction has provoked. Since effort works backward and avoidance is ultimately reinforcing, this therapeutic attitude—one of surrender and nonaction with respect to these observed experiences—is the key to recovery from anticipatory anxiety.

There are three essential components to this shift: They can be summed up in three words: "expect," "accept," and "allow." *Expecting* anticipatory anxiety means understanding that your biology and history have sensitized you and that you are capable of reacting with whooshes of fear and having your imagination hijacked at any time. Expecting is the opposite of hoping you will not be anxious; it prevents you from being blindsided and disappointed when it happens. Denial, head in the sand, or any other type of avoidance is counter to a therapeutic attitude. *Accepting* anticipatory anxiety is acknowledging that you are susceptible to its push toward avoidance and striving toward acknowledging those feelings without regret, resentment, shame, anger, or recrimination. Accepting anxiety includes being willing to experience it. Finally, *allowing* the anxiety is the process of nonaction and therapeutic surrender, which will be addressed in detail in chapter 8. (Please don't skip ahead and read it now—it's better to take first things first.) It means noting the anxiety and its push toward avoidance, leaving it alone, and staying as close to the present as possible while you are anxious. Allowing is a statement of how to be and not what to do.

We cannot emphasize enough that the therapeutic attitude is not a technique for vanquishing anxiety. Remember that any attempt to banish anxiety will not be helpful. You will inadvertently struggle against the feelings, resulting in paradoxical effort, along with the impatience and urgency that goes along with this struggle.

So, what does this mean when we talk about an attitude shift and not a technique? It means a stance to take or a way to be *while* you are observing and experiencing the thoughts and sensations of anxiety. It is not *in order to* make it go away. It is without intention, like sitting on a beach watching the waves, not hoping or trying for any wave to be any different, sooner, or bigger. It is about allowing time to pass while things are as they are.

HELPFUL FACT—The key to recovery lies in changing your attitude toward your thoughts, feelings, memories, sensations, and imagination.

One of the best ways to gain a clearer picture of this process is to introduce "voices of the mind," whose interactions illustrate your challenges and opportunities while you work to overcome anticipatory anxiety and chronic indecision.

Voices of the Mind

If you pay attention to the thoughts that run through your mind, you will see that there are lots of "voices" in your head that dialogue with each other. It is remarkable (and sometimes confusing!) that we often have a variety of thoughts and feelings about the same thing at the same time. Let's look at how two of these voices set up and reinforce both anticipatory anxiety and chronic indecisiveness. In two previous books, we presented three characters who illustrate common internal voices of the mind. Both anticipatory anxiety, and its partner, chronic indecisiveness, are set up, maintained, and made stronger by the interplay between two of these voices. We call these voices Worried Voice and False Comfort. The third voice, which we call Wise Mind, oversees without judgment, provides a metacognitive commentary, and points toward the path to overcoming fearful avoidances.

Worried Voice

Worried Voice is the voice of anticipatory anxiety. Worried Voice comes up with the doubts, the what-ifs, and the "yes, buts." It sets you up to feel anxious and avoidant. Worried Voice is the voice of your frightening overactive imagination. It articulates your fears, doubts, and insecurities. It is persistent and creative. And—this is important—Worried Voice has a very unusual type of memory. If you encounter something one hundred times and have no problem with it ninety-nine times but botch up something or have a bad experience even just one time, guess what experience becomes ingrained in the memory of Worried Voice? Yes, it is the one time it went wrong. Worried Voice will try to never let you forget it! Worried Voice is all or nothing. Either it is good or awful. Catastrophic or perfect. Worried Voice wants guarantees for certainty, safety, and clarity. It wants answers to questions about the future that cannot be answered.

False Comfort

False Comfort wants to hush up Worried Voice. It is the voice of avoidance. The sole purpose of False Comfort is to remove the anxiety that is expressed by Worried Voice. It gets so afraid of the fears and catastrophic rantings of Worried Voice that it constantly tries to argue with, dismiss, reassure, avoid, distract, and make light of Worried Voice. Whenever Worried Voice has a fearful thought, False Comfort comes back with something to try to make that fear go away. False Comfort truly believes that it is helping, trying out various "coping tools," providing rational arguments, or following advice about positive thoughts. It offers "answers" to unanswerable questions. False Comfort comes up with creative ways to try to avoid risk or offers reassurance that can't be backed up—what we often call "empty reassurance."

But here is the problem: No matter how skillfully False Comfort argues, Worried Voice always has a comeback that escalates the anxiety. The ongoing interchange between Worried Voice and False Comfort just ramps up the level of anticipatory anxiety that Worried Voice expresses. Even temporary relief offered by False Comfort backfires.

If you have OCD, you will recognize Worried Voice as anxiety-arousing obsession and False Comfort as *temporary* anxiety-decreasing compulsion.

HELPFUL FACT—Worried Voice is the voice of anticipatory anxiety; False Comfort is the voice of avoidance.

Let's look at how Worried Voice and False Comfort interact when grappling with anticipatory anxiety in a situation that commonly provokes it: giving a presentation at work.

Worried Voice: I just found out that I have to give a presentation in the staff meeting. I am freaking out.

False Comfort: It is not till next week, right? You have plenty of time to prepare. I'm sure you'll do fine.

Worried Voice: It doesn't matter if I write the whole thing out, I am just going to be miserable with anxiety for the whole week. I probably won't sleep, and that will make it worse.

False Comfort: Well, you can take a sleeping pill the night before. And it is just on Zoom, right? So they won't be able to see how nervous you are, even if your hand is shaking.

Worried Voice: But if I read it, I won't be looking into the camera. That always looks weird.

False Comfort: Well, it is only five minutes. Maybe you could memorize it.

Worried Voice: Oh, no! I couldn't do that. I will be so anxious that I'm sure I will forget it. I will be humiliated. I already feel humiliated. What is wrong with me? I have no confidence; I am such a loser.

False Comfort: See, now you are escalating. This always happens. Why don't you just relax and stop thinking about it. You always enjoy watching a good comedy on Netflix.

Worried Voice: I will never be able to concentrate while I feel like this. You're no help. How can I get out of this?

First, let us point out that reading this conversation puts you—the reader—into a metacognitive stance. You are observing the voices of the mind from a "step-back" perspective. And, to the extent that you can identify with them (even if the content may be quite different from your own internal dialogues), you are experiencing the vantage point of metacognition.

You can see how this conversation between Worried Voice and False Comfort never seems to end. False Comfort tries and fails in its effort to silence Worried Voice and, in fact, triggers Worried Voice to come up with additional reasons why it should remain anxious.

This dialogue between Worried Voice and False Comfort illustrates the basic principle that trying to avoid your anxious feelings by comforting yourself in this manner is almost always a mistake—that is why we call it False Comfort. False Comfort often offers typical "coping skills" like analyzing, trying to make an escape plan or a preprepared script, empty reassurance, or experiential or behavioral avoidance strategies. They only work for a moment, and the relief you feel quickly becomes the engine that powers up Worried Voice for yet another round.

There is a distinction that we'd like to make: We have all had the experience of reassuring ourselves about something (*Yes, I do remember locking the door. Come on, I've done this before, I can do it! So what if I buy something I might want to return!*) and then immediately feeling better and proceeding forward. In these cases, it works. However, with anticipatory anxiety, repeated attempts at self-comfort, trying to resolve the issues of doubts and indecision, or trying to rid oneself of the worry just seem to become a spiral of looping and escalating internal arguments.

Remember, it is not the content of the worry thought that counts; it is the way it acts and feels over time: the worry thought repeats and feels awful. Your internal dialogue between Worried Voice and False Comfort is repeatedly entangled in the content of the anticipated catastrophe. *This entanglement—not the content—is the problem.* Being able to step away from content and look at the process is the metacognitive shift that Wise Mind makes.

HELPFUL FACT—Repeated self-comfort (false comfort) almost always results in increased anticipatory anxiety.

Wise Mind

Wise Mind is the way out of the escalating and anxiety-maintaining dialogue between Worried Voice and False Comfort. We all have a Wise Mind, but people who are sensitive to being anxious tend to overlook theirs: it takes some practice to find this voice inside yourself and to listen carefully.

Wise Mind is the voice of plain common sense. It can be sensible even while aware of doubts and worries. It can tolerate acceptable risks and evaluate situations in the real world. It does not get entangled with unwanted intrusive thoughts and flights of imagination, and it can do without constant reassurance. It is a mindful and calm observer of the other internal voices and of the external world and its realities. It knows that doubts are a natural product of the human mind and also that guarantees of health, safety, and success are not possible. It recognizes a likely false alarm when it hears one. Importantly, it does not judge or suppress the other voices and is never critical. It is the one who breaks up unproductive and spiraling anticipatory anxiety by stepping away and refusing to get entangled in a struggle and helps you become unstuck during the times you might feel stuck.

Wise Mind will not—by itself—eliminate your anticipatory anxiety and chronic indecisiveness. It is not trying to alleviate anxiety or doubts. Rather, your own Wise Mind can help you avoid the arguments and missteps that increase your anxiety. This is a point that needs to be made clear. Wise Mind is offering reminders to shift into the therapeutic attitude and to stop struggling. And when you pay attention to Wise Mind, you set the conditions for the other voices to gradually and naturally lose their power to bully you into avoiding actions you wish to take.

> HELPFUL FACT—Wise Mind can point you in the right direction toward overcoming both anticipatory anxiety and chronic indecisiveness but cannot, in itself, eliminate them.

Let's go back to the last part of the dialogue between Worried Voice and False Comfort and see how Wise Mind might inject a measure of good common sense.

False Comfort: See, now you are escalating. This always happens. Why don't you just relax and stop thinking about it? You always enjoy watching a good comedy on Netflix.

Worried Voice: I will never be able to concentrate while I feel like this.

Watch what happens when Wise Mind steps in:

Wise Mind: I can see that this conversation is adding to your anxiety.

False Comfort: I'm trying to help. I don't want Worried Voice to be so frightened. I have to come up with something to relieve the distress.

Wise Mind: I can see that. I can also see that it doesn't seem to be working.

Worried Voice: Yes! Nothing works. My presentation will be a disaster.

Wise Mind: You are trying to fight off anticipatory anxiety. It is not dangerous, only distressing, to feel anxious. Remember that anticipatory imaginings tell you absolutely nothing about how it will actually go. It is not an urgent directive to avoid. You are both falling prey to the false belief that you must relax, prepare better, or change how you feel or else you will fail. Anxious thoughts may be very loud, but they are still thoughts coming from your imagination. There is no help to be had in trying to solve a problem that is a story that Worried Voice is making up.

Worried Voice: But what if my anticipatory anxiety is right?

Wise Mind: The struggle you are having now to try to make yourself feel comfortable is only working backward. When you are feeling so miserable, it is hard to see that empty reassurance and making plans to escape only fuel the doubts. It is actually easier to *expect*, *accept*, and *allow* the feelings of discomfort than to work hard to banish those feelings. Shift your attitude into compassionate observing, not fixing, and you will be able to move forward, with doubts still present.

Worried Voice and False Comfort (together):	You are telling us to stop talking about this, right?
Wise Mind:	Yes. Shift your attention to the present moment, where, in reality, you are in no trouble at all. No need to buy into this scary story. Let the discomfort be what it is, and take your dog out for a walk. She has been scratching at the door for the past fifteen minutes.

Another perspective on this same dialogue is described by the OCD specialist Michael Greenberg (2021). Worried Voice asks, "What if the threat is real, and you ignore it? You will be responsible for a catastrophe." False Comfort is continually asking, "What if the threat is not real, and you are taking it seriously? You will suffer needlessly." Each argues from its own perspective. Worried Voice is worried about false negatives, so it feels compelled to worry, even if the threat is unlikely. False Comfort is always arguing that Worried Voice is suffering from a false positive and should feel reassured and just relax.

Greenberg notes that this dialogue (what we are describing as the commentary of Worried Voice and False Comfort) can be viewed as a court battle between the prosecution and the defense. Worried Voice is the prosecutor, wanting to make absolutely sure that all threats are addressed and even exaggerated—to make the very best case. False Comfort argues for the defense, trying to minimize any accusations hurled by the prosecutor.

To continue with this metaphor, neither Worried Voice (the prosecution) nor False Comfort (the defense) have the perspective of a judge and jury. This is the role of Wise Mind, who can stand back from the argument and realize (like every judge and jury) that there is no way to eliminate uncertainty and that the choice of guilty or not guilty (commit to act or not) must still be made. Wise Mind can identify what is born of creative imagination, rather than the facts in the here and now. It knows what a commonsense best guess decision would be, based on probably, not possibly. Not for sure, but beyond *reasonable* doubt.

Self Study

Choose an example of anticipatory anxiety in your own life right now and try to assign your own internal dialogue voices. See if you can track how they are interacting with each other to escalate your anxiety. Watch the process as they interact, not the content. Try to contact your Wise Mind and step back.

Conclusion

The shift to the therapeutic attitude is so important that we will review the essential elements one more time. We have shown that your former ways of trying to cope with anticipatory anxiety and chronic indecisiveness cannot work. If anything, those methods strengthen the tendency to get hijacked by your imagination. However, as you switch your awareness to a nonjudgmental, metacognitive perspective, you are in the position to disentangle yourself from the scary content of your imagination and observe the process that keeps anxiety alive. The therapeutic attitude is letting go of the struggle: "Wait, you can't fight this. That only makes it worse. You are being beaten up by your imagination." Here is where your good common sense enters in the form of your own Wise Mind with the perspective to say, "These choices are worthwhile. You might feel anxiety, but delaying and avoiding will only keep you stuck. Instead, moving toward the uncomfortable feelings, embracing them, and surrendering to them is the way out of this anxiety trap." The three words that embody this attitude are "expect," "accept," and "allow."

In the next chapter, we will explore how to make this shift and move forward.

CHAPTER 8

Surrender and Commit:
The Antidote to Avoidance

In earlier chapters, we introduced anticipatory anxiety and chronic indecisiveness, showed you the various ways that they present themselves, and explained how your brain and body can get hijacked by your imagination. We addressed the important concepts of anxiety sensitivity, sticky mind, paradoxical effort, and negative reinforcement. Understanding these concepts—and how they apply to your anticipatory anxiety—begins the process of learning to recognize when your imagination takes over and to stop doing the things that make it so difficult for you to move forward in the face of this anxiety. In chapter 7, we introduced two essential concepts: the metacognitive perspective, which allows you to disentangle from the content of your thoughts, and the therapeutic attitude, which can be summed up by the words "expect," "accept," and "allow."

Important Note. For many who are suffering, there is the temptation to skip over the "descriptive" parts of self-help books and turn to the "what to do" chapters right away. If you have started reading here, we hope that you go back to the beginning of this book. These next chapters will not be as helpful without the context of the detailed explanations we have laid out as groundwork.

For all forms of anxiety, exposure is an active, therapeutic, brain-rewiring ingredient. To gain confidence and learn from experience, you will be making decisions and moving forward *while* you are feeling anxious. Conquering anticipatory anxiety will include putting yourself in situations that trigger at least some anxiety, learning each time how to handle the experience. At the same time, you will also be learning to stay connected to the therapeutic attitude, noting from a metacognitive perspective where your Worried Voice and False Comfort dialogues lead you astray.

You have probably tried to overcome your anticipatory anxiety in the past, and—if you are reading this book—your efforts have been far less successful than you had hoped. So why should it be different this time? Why should you yet again put yourself through the pain of moving toward your anxiety? The answer is that while you might have worked very hard in the past and your efforts might very well have been heroic, they were probably misplaced. *There was nothing wrong with you, your effort, or your energy, but there was most likely something very wrong with your approach.*

> HELPFUL FACT—There is nothing wrong with you, just the methods and attitudes you have been using.

This new approach is far more effective and long-lasting and gives you the very best chance of changing your patterns of avoidance and indecision. You already understand that effort works backward when you're trying to cope with anxiety, and that avoidance—both behavioral and experiential—reinforces anxiety in the longer term. So, let's get on with a discussion of applying this perspective and attitude as you experience anticipatory imaginings. We'll pay particular attention to avoiding the detours created by your inner anxious dialogues. And then we will explore the role that commitment plays in exposure: exposure done with commitment is effective. Exposure without the change in perspective and attitude is often forced and painful and usually backfires.

Recovering Begins with Perspective and Attitude Shifts

Recovering begins with a commitment to noticing when your what-if thought gets amplified by your imagination into an anxiety-generating story and when you respond involuntarily to that story. So, for example, if you plan to face a challenge next week and your Worried Voice pops up with "What if I mess up?" a metacognitive perspective allows you to say, "I'm noticing myself anxiously reacting to that thought." There will be a great pull by your creative imagination to continue that story and for you to react with even greater anxiety as you elaborate upon and react to the images you create. This pull to elaborate can be very compelling.

This is the point where you begin to leave your own good common sense—your own Wise Mind—and enter the world of your imagination. Remember that there is a fact-based world that goes: "I am meeting a challenge tomorrow, and I am anxious about it." Those are the facts. Additionally, there is the world of your imagination, which creates a story that we call "anticipatory imaginings." This creates the specter of anticipatory anxiety.

This commitment encompasses a shift in two aspects of your relationship with your inner experience: a shift in perspective and a shift in attitude.

Shifting perspective has two components:

1. A hands-off, observational approach to your emotional life

2. Valuing the present moment

Shifting attitude has three components:

1. A nonjudgmental, self-compassionate stance

2. Willingness: a leaning toward rather than away from anxiety-challenging experiences

3. Therapeutic surrender

We are now going to take a closer look at these five components of changing your relationship with your inner experience.

Watch but Don't Touch

Observing and labeling your anxious thought as it occurs is an important step to halt the hijacking of your imagination. It is the first step in the shift to a metacognitive perspective. Let's suppose that you are driving over a bridge tomorrow, and think, *What if I panic and drive off the bridge?* You might note your thoughts in the following way: *I'm having an anxious thought, I'm feeling a whoosh of fear, and my heart is beating rapidly.*

> HELPFUL FACT—Observe with no intention to engage or change.

You might have realized that we are not asking you to address the *content* of your thoughts. You are only noticing that they are raising (or lowering) your anxiety, and—in the case of worry thoughts—that they seem to keep repeating. This is an example of staying connected to the process of your awareness, as opposed to the content.

Anticipatory anxiety is one of those times in life when doing anything makes things worse. This is when doing less is more and doing nothing is best. Observe your inner life, your anxious feelings, the sensations in your body, and your memories of the past, but don't engage with them. This hands-off perspective can be easily misunderstood, so let's look at it more closely.

If I have the Worried Voice thought, *What if I have a panic attack when I take the train?* then engaging with the thought involves some sort of response to that thought. Here is an example: If I then think, *Don't worry, it won't be so bad* (False Comfort), I am responding to the thought, reassuring myself, and inadvertently reinforcing the original what-if thought. Instead, a nonengaged Wise Mind perspective might say, "I'm having a thought that is making me anxious." This approach acknowledges your thought and the anxiety that automatically arises from it but doesn't get entangled with it, thereby depriving your alarm system of the fuel it needs in order to escalate.

If I think to myself, *Oh no, I remember the last time I took a train, and I had the awful panic attack that ruined my whole day. What if it happens again?* A nonengaged response would note that my old memory has triggered anticipatory anxiety.

In past chapters, we described the three concepts of (1) paradoxical effort, (2) the anxiety reinforcement that results from avoidance, and (3) the fact that struggling to quell anxiety ultimately leads to more anxiety. When you address the content of your thoughts, it becomes almost impossible not to engage with your doubts and worries. That is why we focus on simply observing what is happening without addressing what seems like an "issue" or a "problem."

There is a common misunderstanding of mindfulness that needs clarification. It is not helpful to be mindful of False Comfort ruminations. "Mindfully" following along as you continue your dialogue with Worried Voice ("I am aware of devising an escape plan. I am aware of offering an argument for avoidance. I am aware of trying to get Worried Voice to relax.") is certainly not helpful. Here is what is helpful: refrain from offering false comfort at all; instead, shift into the present moment and disentangle yourself from the inner dialogue, as your own observing Wise Mind reminds you to do.

HELPFUL FACT—It is most helpful not to offer any false comfort at all.

In the same way, simply observing your feelings—*I am anxious, I am disgusted, I am ashamed*—is all we are talking about. It is not, as some suggest, "mindfully" thinking about, dwelling upon, disputing, "meditating about," or in any way exploring these feelings. It is not helpful to ask why at this point. Just stand back and be aware. Simply observing happens without the intent to change anything.

HELPFUL FACT—It is almost never helpful to ask why when you are anxious.

To hope that mindfulness alone will effect a desired change is also a misunderstanding. The metacognitive shift to mindful awareness is a prerequisite for change—it does not by itself create change.

Worried Voice: I can't bear the thought that my baby could get sick.

False Comfort: She is a perfect little baby; there is nothing to worry about.

Worried Voice: But you can't guarantee that she will be fine forever. I imagine being helpless to protect her, then she dies, and then I can never recover.

False Comfort: Maybe you could say a prayer every day to keep her safe. That would feel better. Why are you even thinking this now?

Wise Mind: How about just acknowledge that you had a painful thought. There is nothing to be gained by thinking about that thought or how to deal with it. Let it be.

Value the Present

Anxiety lives in the future. Whether your anxiety is triggered by odd sensations, frightening thoughts, or scary memories, the process of imagining the what-if future is what keeps your alarm system going and turns temporary whooshes of anxiety into ongoing anticipatory anxiety. Most anxious people are surprised to realize how little time they spend attending to the present.

When you notice that you are stuck in your imagined future, focus on what is rather than what if: this means gently dislodge yourself from your Worried Voice and return to the reality you are actually in right now. When we are anxious, we are hypervigilant, having inadvertently trained our brains to be on the lookout for dangers in this situation. The most effective way to return to the present moment is to leave the arena of thinking and instead pay attention to your senses—the background sounds as you read this book, the sensations in your legs as you sit in the chair, and the texture of the paper in your hands (or the feel of the e-reader). Be aware of your sensory experiences as they change from moment to moment. Here, in this very moment, nothing bad is happening to you in reality, there is no external urgency, and your thoughts about the future can retreat in favor of what you see and hear and sense right now. You don't have to DO anything, just BE. Let time pass. To (incorrectly) paraphrase the Beatles, "Let it be, let it be, [there's no need to answer], let it be."

It is important to be clear about a distinction that can seem tricky. It concerns both intention and attention when you shift from what-if to what is. The goal is to gently turn your attention back to the present moment. It is not in order to try *to suppress, banish, or ignore* the worried script so it will go away. Instead, *while* you are aware of those anticipatory imaginings, simply turn toward your present sensory experience. *It is a shift of attention, without intention.*

HELPFUL FACT—Attend to what is instead of what if.

When we clarify the distinction between what if and what is, it becomes clear that thinking about something is the defining factor in leaving the present: the issue is initiated by imaginative, scary thoughts. In a nutshell, *anticipatory anxiety is all about too much thinking. And too much thinking is not solved with more thinking.* It is precisely when you notice that you are engaged with your internal Worried Voice–False Comfort dialogue that Wise Mind can encourage you to leave the argument and gently return to the present moment. When avoidance may seem like the best option, when you are frustrated by being so stuck, when you are bargaining with yourself for some way out, or when you are busy weaving tales about potential catastrophes, commit to stepping back from your thoughts and return to value the present. This is a very simple suggestion. You will notice, if you let a little time pass and you let it register that there is no real emergency right now, that your overactive alarm system subsides.

HELPFUL FACT—Problems related to too much thinking are not solved with more thinking.

It is difficult to remain immersed in your imagination while simultaneously attending to your senses in the present moment. This is because sensory pathways and imagination pathways in the brain are different circuits. Although sensory information does not block or stop creative story-making about the future, stepping back and adding a sensory focus to your experience (the temperature of your breath, the sounds you hear, the wrinkles of your knuckles, the pressure of the chair against your back) interrupts that compulsive desire to keep thinking about, expanding on, elaborating on, and responding to the anxious imaginings.

Worried Voice: This meal reminds me that I am having guests next week. I am worried about being the host. I have to plan the meal, cook, clean the whole place, and still make sure everyone has a good time.

False Comfort: There is nothing to be worried about. You always do it well.

Worried Voice: But my schedule is so busy, and I worry that I have lost my touch for cooking.

False Comfort: You could have it catered. And plan some kind of game for people to play.

Worried Voice: That won't work. People expect me to cook. And games are silly. What am I going to do? I won't sleep for a week. How can I entertain if I feel this panicky now?

False Comfort: You could always tell people you have your "migraine."

Worried Voice: I can't stand how I am.

Wise Mind: I can see from over here that you are both scrambling to solve a problem that has not happened and is only in your mind. Every suggestion is some way to avoid and makes things worse. How about slowing down and paying attention to the taste of the meal you are presently eating, instead of the imagined burned catastrophic meal in your imagination? That pasta sauce could use some salt.

We understand that no one can live entirely in the moment. We all have to plan our day, get the kids ready for school, schedule the doctor appointment, take in the car for service, prepare for the trip, and find enough time to shop, cook, and maybe fit in a visit to the gym. It is said that living entirely in the moment is a great life for a golden retriever puppy, but not so great for adult humans! Still, there is room in virtually everyone's life to both plan their day and value the ability to attend to the present.

Nonjudgmental Self-Compassion

Remaining nonjudgmental is an essential part of the attitude shift. This is sometimes confusing for our patients. The most common response goes something like "I need to be hard on myself. It is my self-discipline and self-control that gets me through the day and keeps me from falling apart entirely!"

Committing to a nonjudgmental attitude has nothing to do with sloppiness or lack of discipline in learning to overcome your anticipatory anxiety. Rather, it is about committing to the compassionate observation of the way you react to triggers and the ways in which you automatically tend to judge yourself. This is not about doing anything differently in the external world—but we are asking that you change the way you judge your actions and reactions in your *internal* world. To be specific, self-compassion is *not* about giving yourself permission to avoid whenever you are feeling anxious or distressed. It is not about "letting yourself off the hook." It is about feeling kindness about your pain or worry—and offering support for your bravery and strength in the face of doubts and fears. *Nonjudgmental self-compassion is always about valuing who you are at your core, rather than about what you accomplish.*

When you fail to note an anxious thought, get caught up in the content of your worries, or get stuck in looping internal dialogue, allow yourself to step away without self-reproach or frustrated self-criticism. When you catch yourself resorting to old, ineffectual ways of coping with anxiety, note that nonjudgmentally as well. Do your best to be patient with yourself. This takes practice.

We firmly believe that there is room for both discipline and self-compassion. You can work as hard as you can—be utterly committed—and still find room to be gentle with yourself when (not if, but when) you notice that you have fallen short of your goals. And when you are unable to be gentle with yourself in these situations, note that as well. Gently bring yourself back to the nonjudgmental present—and keep on going.

Willingness

Willingness is the attitude of leaning toward anxiety-producing events and decisions instead of hoping to avoid them. Commitment to this attitude is based on the belief that distress and discomfort are not truly dangerous and that the path to recovery lies through them, not around them. Willingness is about allowing your mind and body to experience the anxiety whether it is in the form of harmless sensations of arousal, clanging false alarms, or frightened imaginings that keep popping up. It is about willingly focusing on having the experience so you can rewire your brain, rather than trying to not have the experience. It is about long-term gain rather than short-term relief.

The attitude of willingness is the opposite of white-knuckling (holding your breath, hoping to avoid anxiety, plowing through by counting off the time). It is about withdrawing efforts to control what you feel and simply observing what is happening. Willingness requires an understanding of how anxiety is triggered and maintained. Decreasing anxiety in the long term often requires the willingness to accept greater distress in the short term.

Willingness is not a natural stance. Running away from or avoiding perceived danger is hardwired. It takes being committed to your recovery to willingly approach what you fear. But once you enter an attitude of willingness, you will discover how it works. The panic you willingly allow is much less likely because you have abandoned your typical exertion of overcontrol. When you are not braced for a blow, you respond more flexibly. And change starts to happen.

One patient with a long-standing fear of heights demonstrates her commitment to willingness by always answering "yes" whenever someone asks her to meet at the top of a tall building to share a drink or enjoy the view. She sometimes comments, "Well, there is a view, but I'm not sure how much I'm enjoying it. But it does get easier."

HELPFUL FACT—Long-term anxiety reduction often requires a willingness to accept greater anxiety in the short term.

Worried Voice: I want to visit my grandmother, but she is on the thirty-seventh floor. No way am I going to climb those stairs again. I nearly gave myself a heart attack.

False Comfort: Why can't you ride the elevator? They all have those emergency phones in them.

Worried Voice: I have had panic attacks on elevators. That is way too much cardiac stress.

False Comfort: I know you can do it. Just close your eyes and count to one hundred. You'll be there in no time. Or maybe the concierge could go with you? You know the doctor says that you don't have cardiac issues.

Worried Voice: And what if the elevator gets stuck? And, even if I made it to my grandmother, I would be freaked-out the whole time because I would have to go back down. Not worth it.

False Comfort: I see what you mean. Zoom is a good substitute.

Worried Voice: She is so disappointed in me. She is eighty-one, and she can ride elevators. Makes me feel terrible.

False Comfort: You are a good person; it is not your fault. Don't go. She will forgive you.

Wise Mind: See how you are letting your anticipatory anxiety run your life? Your false belief—that a panic attack is unendurable—is robbing you of the pleasure of seeing her. The more you struggle to come up with some way to avoid the anxiety, the more upset you become. How about committing to practicing being anxious on a shorter elevator trip a few times? Then you will be more willing to be anxious. You could also hope for a panic attack so you could practice simply allowing time to pass while your body settles down on its own. Remember "expect," "accept," and "allow"? Your body's false alarm is unpleasant but worth your freedom.

Therapeutic Surrender

When we tell patients that the path to recovery lies through the attitude of surrender, they say "What?" in surprise and disappointment. "So the key to recovery is to give up? Like I'm going to have to endure this anxiety forever and never get over it? Why can't you just give me better coping skills?" And we reply, "This has nothing to do with giving up. But when you realize that most of your anguish comes from your attempt to fight anxiety and that your avoidance interferes with building new neural pathways, you will see that the most effective way forward is to change your relationship with your anxiety so it can no longer run your life or tell you what to do." This is the attitude of therapeutic surrender, the third component of the attitude shift necessary to change your relationship with your inner experience. It is a more profound and lasting change than that which any coping skills can give you.

Therapeutic surrender simply means abandoning the struggle. It is the struggle that creates paradoxical effort and desperate avoidance measures and keeps you stuck in the escalating Worried Voice and False Comfort dialogues. Imagine you are in a tug-of-war with your anxiety. It has the strength to pull you forward, and then, with every bit of your energy, you can pull it back toward the middle. But the game never ends, and no one can win because you are equally matched. The struggle is forever. Now step back and imagine this: right while your opponent is pulling the hardest, you drop the rope and refuse to play. Anxiety will tumble backward and fall down (Harris 2017). *Therapeutic surrender is a refusal to play anxiety's game.*

This means staying close to your Wise Mind, who embodies a refusal to play, refrains from being hijacked by your imagination, and steps away from the false narratives you are spinning about disastrous outcomes. The attitude of therapeutic surrender lets you stay connected to your common sense. And by not buying into your catastrophic thinking and imagined dangers, but instead by refusing to treat doubts as facts or predictions, it is easier to make the commitment to proceed. This allows you to undertake the experiences that can teach your brain and body to be less reactive when confronted with a challenge.

Therapeutic surrender means surrendering control; trusting that you will handle whatever thoughts, sensations, and feelings happen; and allowing your body and mind to right themselves naturally with the passage of time. It takes a leap of faith to surrender—you will commit to a decision or an action with no guarantees that it will go well. But surrender removes the fuel that powers the anxiety because you are withdrawing from the struggle.

Imagine that you are driving a car—a strange car—one that is equipped with a gas pedal but no brake. You are speeding along a flat road out in a desert and decide you want to stop. You could reach for the brake, find it is missing, and flail about the car in a panic, accidentally stepping on the gas repeatedly. You might even swerve off the road, leading to other consequences even more dire. Or you could simply surrender: take your foot off the gas, do nothing except let time pass, and wait while the car slowly runs out of gas and drifts to a safe stop, further down the road.

Here is an example of Wise Mind stepping in to recommend therapeutic surrender as Worried Voice and False Comfort are stuck in an endless loop.

Worried Voice: I want to buy a hybrid car, but I keep changing my mind about which one is best. I am driving myself and everyone around me nuts.

False Comfort: Why don't you check the ratings?

Worried Voice: Don't you think I have? But I can't go by them because only people with raves and beefs bother to rate.

False Comfort: How about an objective rating by a car website?

Worried Voice: There are new ones popping up every day. I am monitoring eleven of them. They say different things.

False Comfort: Why don't you delay till there is a consensus on next year's models?

Worried Voice: Delay again this year? My car is falling apart.

False Comfort: Well, just toss a coin then.

Worried Voice: But I will never live it down if I pick wrong or pay too much. I will be mortified.

Wise Mind: This is getting nowhere. Round and round. You are letting your anticipatory imaginings about regret bully you. You will need to be willing to make a less-than-perfect choice here. You might have regrets of some kind, but at least you will have a car. Make a choice, and then, before you have time to reconsider it again, commit to the sale online or in person—and hand over your credit card or sign the documents. There will be a surge of feelings after that. Ride them out and do nothing more.

Now that we have described the perspective and attitude shifts that are requisites for learning new ways to approach anticipatory anxiety, we will show you how to implement these in your daily life.

DANCE: The Five Steps of Therapeutic Surrender

There are five steps to applying the perspective and attitude that help you overcome both anxiety and chronic indecisiveness. We have already gone over all the specifics, and now we are going to show you how to practice moving forward in this different way. Here is an easy way to remember it: DANCE. It is a convenient reminder that moving forward is about gently dancing with anxiety, not fighting for control. This practice is *how to be* each time as you naturally encounter anticipatory anxiety in your life.

D: Discern your anticipatory anxiety as imagination, memory, sensitization, or mood, and disentangle yourself.

A: Accept doubts and discomfort willingly.

N: No struggling, avoiding, reassuring, or overthinking.

C: Commit to proceed with action or choice.

E: Embrace the present as it is and let time pass.

DANCE can be applied with equal effectiveness to both anticipatory anxiety and chronic indecisiveness. Don't try to apply the steps too rigidly. Dance with them; don't make it a march! Rather, allow for a flexible and fluid visit to each of these steps whenever they are needed. Let's take a closer look at each of the components.

D: Discern your anticipatory anxiety as imagination, memory, sensitization, or mood, and disentangle yourself. You experience an immediate thought, desire, or need to take action. Almost concurrently, you feel a whoosh of arousal, and anticipatory anxiety begins. It is a familiar feeling you recognize. *This is your cue to zoom out to a metacognitive perspective.*

This is part of a pattern in your life, not a unique event. You might notice a disturbing worry thought or a memory of past fear that is elaborated by your imagination. You may be aware that your mood, recent stressors, or particular triggers are contributing to your distress. Be aware of the pull to avoid. Notice how your anxiety increases as you weave a story in your imagination about the future. *Discerning is not an invitation to do anything other than mindfully observe.*

A: Accept doubts and discomfort willingly. Expect, allow, and accept is the advice of your Wise Mind. Doubts arise automatically: *Is this the right choice? Will I be able to handle the consequences if I am wrong? What if my anxiety gets too high—maybe I should cancel?* You feel unwelcome uncertainty. Your body feels the discomfort of arousal. These are not warnings or predictions. The doubts have no real power. You have been here before.

As you look from a disentangled perspective—the view from a distance—remind yourself to observe the process you have recognized, and do not get immersed in the details of this particular challenge. It will be helpful now to ask yourself if you are still in touch with your Wise Mind, and if not, at what point did you lose your common sense and get hijacked by your imagination? *This is about shifting your attitude from resistance to willingness.*

N: No struggling, avoiding, reassuring, or overthinking. Struggling against discomfort may be the natural stance, but you know that effort works backward, and the less you do, the more productive your practice becomes. In the same light, avoidance, self-reassurance, and trying to plan how to cope are natural but only work temporarily. Overthinking and ruminating about the details of this specific challenge do nothing but lead you into more looping worries. *This is a reminder to let it be.*

C: Commit to proceed with action or choice. Undertake your challenge while being aware of feeling anxious: do not wait for confidence or the right moment or a feeling of being sure. Commit to some step forward, even if small, no matter how you feel. Don't be tentative and don't plan your escape. Do not be tricked by your imagination into thinking your anticipatory distress is a signal of danger or fragility or disability. A meta-cognitive perspective and willing attitude make commitment possible. Oscillating indecision and lack of commitment make it worse. *This is a reminder that making a firm commitment makes it better.*

E: Embrace the present as it is and let time pass. While you are proceeding toward what you fear, whether it is making a choice or undertaking an activity, shift your attention away from the doubting, worrying what-ifs of Worried Voice and the avoiding, struggling, reassuring attempts of False Comfort. Instead, move toward the present reality—to the experience of what is. There is no emergency in the present moment. This is not intended to banish your anticipatory anxiety: it is how to be while you allow time to pass and allow anxiety to diminish on its own. *This is a reminder to gently shift away from thinking toward sensing.*

Practicing DANCE in Daily Life

Once you understand DANCE and have applied it a few times, it is time to practice. In the same way that you can't learn to dance by just reading about it, you must practice these steps in your daily life until they become natural. Commit to lean into and seize every opportunity to build new experiences and assist your brain to create new circuitry. Don't pick and choose. Just do what comes next, whatever challenges present themselves in the normal flow of your life. Welcome each decision point or new activity as a chance to practice. Your progress will surprise you if you make this commitment.

> HELPFUL FACT—Just like learning to dance, learning DANCE takes practicing the steps.

If someone asks you to attend an event and you get that whoosh, step out to mindful awareness, notice how you are creating fearful imaginings, lean in willingly, and commit to going—no matter how strong the pull to avoid. If you have to see the doctor, notice yourself remembering the anxious week before the last visit, remind yourself this is an opportunity to learn what it is like to accept and allow anxious arousal and commit to a specific appointment time. If you have to file your taxes, commit to the time to do it, check your work only once, and submit the forms. Then expect and allow the immediate whoosh caused by automatic doubts. Let time pass.

If you are juggling two job offers and might lose both if you don't act, drop the dialogue between Worried Voice and False Comfort, step back from the struggle, and ask your Wise Mind. You may already know what to do. If you can't choose which tie to wear, remember it is not about ties—it is about uncertainty. Quickly lay out a few on your bed and commit with your eyes closed.

Worried Voice:	If I am this anxious now, how will I survive next week? I need to prepare!
False Comfort:	We survived before; we'll make a plan. We can back out if we have to.
Wise Mind:	The answer here is not to offer empty reassurance or avoidance, but to commit without guarantees and to stop this struggle. Withdraw control and let time pass. You are stronger than you think. You can do this.

Committing to Planned-Exposure Practice

Up to now, we have addressed shifting your perspective and attitude when you are naturally confronted with choice points or undertaking an activity that triggers anticipatory anxiety. We call this type of practice "incidental practice" because your practice is incidental to the choices and situations that naturally occur in your life. There is yet another step to take in order to make your recovery last: the *intentional* undertaking of choices and anxiety-producing actions that don't present themselves as immediate challenges. Why on earth would anyone deliberately expose themselves to anxious distress if they don't have to? you might ask. Because these experiences are how the brain learns to be less anxious. And the more of them the better.

How to Practice Planned Exposure

Exposure is often called the "active therapeutic ingredient." In the past, terms such as "desensitization," "habituation," and "extinction" were used to describe aspects of this process. Today, inhibitory learning theory accounts for the most contemporary understanding of how it works. This theory states that repeated exposure, done with the right attitude, creates new inhibitory circuitry in the brain, and eventually these new pathways override the former automatic anxious ones (Craske et al. 2014).

But exposure is not an automatic path to recovery. If performed incorrectly, exposure can lead to misery, hopelessness, and even more sensitization. "Just do it" is not helpful advice. We have shown that the DANCE approach encompasses the elements needed to practice during incidental exposure. DANCE is also applicable to planned exposure, which involves intentionally setting up exposure tasks that do not arise on their own, creating additional opportunities to practice. Planned DANCE exposure is most effective when certain guidelines are followed. These include manageability, a focus on the correct triggers, avoiding avoidances, variability, and a commitment to the therapeutic attitude. Let's take a look at each of these guidelines.

Exposure needs to be manageable. Your goal is to move toward rather than away from what makes you anxious, *to treat anticipatory anxiety as the illusion that it is*. However, the attitude of willingness to be uncomfortable does not mean that you must throw yourself directly and precipitously at the very thing that scares you the most. You will do better when you push yourself—*but not to the point that you lose the ability to mindfully observe your distress*. On the other hand, decisions that are too easy or activities that do not challenge you at all are not learning experiences for your brain.

> HELPFUL FACT—Treat anticipatory anxiety as the illusion that it is.

The best learning is empowering: it gives you the confidence and awareness of self-resources to do more of what you value and what matters to you. This applies to any choice or situation whether or not you experience anxiety as you proceed. Keep this in mind as you practice exposure to anxiety triggering events. There is no formula like "baby steps" or any rigid hierarchy of exposures to do. It is more important that you pick something that matters, something that challenges but does not utterly overwhelm you as you imagine it, and something you can commit to doing willingly, allowing whatever thoughts, sensations, feelings, and memories show up.

> HELPFUL FACT—The best planned exposures are stretches that still allow for mindful self-observation.

Exposure has to focus on the correct triggers. This can seem confusing at times. In general, triggers do not refer to a particular physical situation or activity. Anticipatory anxiety is a product of the imagination, so it very well may be a thought or an image that is the trigger. If you have had past anxious experiences when eating in a restaurant, the next reservation might trigger the thought *What if it happens again?* This is the trigger—the worry thought—you want to target, not the restaurant or even eating in the restaurant. Set up a restaurant experience for next week that is *likely* to create anticipatory anxious arousal, one that includes the specific conditions you worry about, whether it is feeling trapped, having to choose from the menu, eating with someone specific, or worrying about being fatigued.

One way to figure out what to expose yourself to is to target whatever you wish to avoid. If it is the experience of feeling uncertain, the exposure is to doubts and maybes. While acknowledging that you're feeling anxious and uncertain, proceed with some deliberately selected valued action, even without the guarantee. Make a choice without much research or deliberation. If it is the possibility of making a mistake, do something and then do not check your work. If you are hoping to avoid regrets, acknowledge that regrets could happen and make the decision anyway. If you want to avoid feeling trapped, target the experience of feeling trapped. If your anticipatory anxiety is about the fear that you will not be able to handle that feeling, will need to run away, and will be unable to do so, find a way to experience feeling trapped, whether it is an elevator, a closet in your home, a traffic jam, or a social "trap," such as a meeting.

Avoiding avoidances makes exposure effective. This is the absolutely essential N of DANCE (no avoidance). Planned exposure is about deliberately setting yourself up to feel anticipatory anxiety. As soon as you do, you will feel the automatic pull toward avoidance, bargaining, self-reassuring, arguing, and ruminating. Even subtle experiential avoidance undermines exposure. It may be useful to go back and look at the list of common overt and more subtle avoidance behaviors in chapter 4. As you willingly and deliberately head toward the experience of anxiety, the awareness of uncertainty, and the knowledge that there are no guarantees to be had, you will feel a pull to make it easier by distracting, limiting, escape planning, or any other safety behaviors you have used in the past to get by. You may even have been taught in therapy or through other self-help books to use some of these behaviors as "coping skills." This is because they do, in fact, temporarily lower the anxiety level. However, we now know that ultimately these kinds of behaviors backfire, serve as negative reinforcers, and do not contribute to building new brain circuitry to make it easier in the long run.

Variability increases effectiveness. Challenge yourself by setting up situations that will evoke anticipatory anxiety in many different arenas. Choose a commitment to something you will do today and something that is planned for next month. Vary the degree of feeling trapped, vulnerable, or disgusted that you expect to face. Challenge your imagination to make up different kinds of stories for you to refuse to buy in to. Deliberately evoke a memory of something you did last week—or a decade ago—that will reliably provoke anxious uncertainty about its consequences. Make different kinds of decisions without checking or excessive research. This variation—in both imagined intensity of anxiety and how far in the future you plan—boosts the creation of new brain pathways (Sewart and Craske 2020).

Commit to the therapeutic attitude as well as to the exposure. Even a rock-solid commitment to exposure may not be helpful if it is done with the wrong attitude. Exposure well done need not be a wrestling match in which you are trying to do something challenging while simultaneously trying to force yourself not to have doubts, remain calm, and hold on to a "get over it" attitude. There must be self-compassion about and willingness toward feeling anxious. Remember to proceed not based on how you feel at the time, but on what you committed to when you planned the practice. Anticipatory anxiety will try to trick you into thinking you can't do it. This is why commitment is incredibly empowering.

DANCE Toward Recovery

While you intentionally lean toward anticipating actions and decisions that cause you anxiety, revisit each of the steps whenever you notice you are struggling, white-knuckling, avoiding, or engaging in Worried Voice–False Comfort ruminating dialogues. Be kind to yourself internally but remain firmly committed to moving forward while actively allowing the presence of anticipatory anxious discomfort of mind and body. Gently remind yourself to commit and surrender while feeling doubts and refusing to play anxiety's game. Freedom is on the other side of this practice.

Self Study

Spend the next few days observing your life for opportunities to apply DANCE in incidental practice. Choose to move toward anxiety whenever the urge to avoid shows up. As you become more familiar with and understand the attitude and perspective shifts we are describing, create some planned-exposure situations to practice further and consolidate what you are learning.

Conclusion

You are gaining the knowledge and mindset to view each challenge as part of a larger process. If you struggle with chronic indecisiveness, you are now seeing how to practice committing to choices as part of your everyday life. If you suffer from anticipatory anxiety, you are learning to recognize the many subtle (and not so subtle) avoidances that have become so automatic. Then, you can challenge yourself to let them go.

Neither anticipatory anxiety nor chronic indecisiveness need be viewed as a series of individual battles with anxiety. As your brain learns, the shift in perspective is facilitated. The steps of DANCE become more natural, flowing together as a simple shift in your relationship with yourself, your body, and your mind whenever you are anxious or stuck.

In the next chapter, we answer common questions that arise as you undertake your journey to recovery.

CHAPTER 9

Troubleshooting: Common Questions Answered

In this chapter, we address some of the confusions and frustrations that typically show up while learning to make the necessary attitudinal, perspective, and behavioral shifts on your path to recovery. It is to be expected that you will get stuck and find yourself mired in old unproductive patterns, even after expending lots of energy and effort. You may be trying with the best of intentions, but your energy and effort can easily be unwittingly misdirected.

The most important message is that of self-compassion and patience: changing lifelong habits of the body and mind takes time, effort, repetition, and the ability to learn from missteps. In fact, those times when you swerve off course are the very best times to learn something new. Here are some of the most common themes of questions we receive.

Question—*I have terrible anticipatory anxiety when I have to drive outside my neighborhood. I have to do a "dry run" with my husband the day before so I know exactly what I am facing. And even then, I am still unable to sleep the night before. How can I do better? Can you give me a step-by-step plan for decreasing my anticipatory anxiety?*

Answer—You have already taken the first step here, by acknowledging that the way you are dealing with your anticipatory anxiety is not working. There are clues in your question. The desire to know "exactly" what you are facing is understandable, but that certainty is impossible to establish even if you do a dry run. It does not stop your what-if imagining as you lie in bed the night before. The key here is to practice *not* knowing for sure exactly what you are facing, first with something small and then building your flexibility and willingness to rely on your own resources in the moment.

Here's one of many options. Pick a place to find on your own, just outside your neighborhood. Make it a low-stakes kind of practice: there's no issue of how long it takes to get there, there's nothing to be late for, there's no assignment to find a place to park, it's okay to use the GPS in the car. But do it on your own. Notice how you feel the pull of avoidance, the discomfort of whatever you imagine might go wrong. Stay committed to going no matter how you feel.

After this, plan more practices and gradually increase the difficulty on different dimensions. Include more things you can't know for sure, such as where to park and more time, to get through before you allow yourself to go. Add in a phone call to be made by a certain time from the place you have found. Increase the distance outside your comfort zone. Keep noticing all the ways your mind and body try to provide false comfort. And give yourself points for the willingness to be uncomfortable while you anticipate each task you have assigned yourself. Practice the perspective and attitude of DANCE as you expect, accept, and allow whatever your mind and body are doing while you move through your exposure to uncertainty, the possibility of messing up, and the chance that you will not be able to do it. Remember that the growth happens when you commit and follow through, not whether you end up being anxious or not. Take a victory lap for each practice you do.

It does not always get easier in a straight line. There are ups and downs and unexpected detours. It takes repetition to learn how to surrender to the experience instead of struggling and trying to avoid being anxious in whatever way you are used to. But gradually you will notice that it is the firm commitment to do it that helps.

Question—*I never avoid doing the things I have anticipatory anxiety about, but no matter how many times I practice, it never gets easier. No matter what I do to distract myself, I am riveted on how anxious I feel, and I can't overcome it. I talk to myself all the time, telling myself I will be okay, but it doesn't work. No matter how much I talk to myself, my irrational self always wins over my rational self.*

Answer—First, congratulations for your courage and commitment! You deserve a huge amount of credit. But sometimes both courage and commitment aren't enough, and it must be frustrating to work so hard and see no results.

It sounds like you are doing what we call "white-knuckling." This keeps your anxiety alive because of paradoxical effort—trying with all your heart, energy, and commitment, but trying in a way that isn't helpful. All the things you do to try to feel better actually keep your anxiety up and make you feel that each experience is just another ordeal to get through. If you could look at each episode of anticipatory anxiety as a learning experience, you'll be able to handle ensuing episodes more effectively.

You describe a number of safety behaviors you are using. Remember that they might make the experience more manageable in the short term, but they keep your anticipatory anxiety alive. You try to distract yourself and give yourself empty reassurance. This is not a struggle between rationality and irrationality: the way forward is not to struggle at all. Look back at the conversations between Worried Voice and False Comfort. Remember that these go nowhere, and your task is to find your own Wise Mind. It is the attitude of surrender, and specifically the *willingness* to experience discomfort in the moment (and to leave it alone, not try to fix it), that is the missing ingredient. Without this willingness, your exposure efforts predictably do not result in therapeutic learning.

Choosing to face your fears instead of avoiding them is very important indeed. But the most therapeutic exposures occur when you can maintain both the perspective of mindful self-observation and the attitude of surrender.

Question—*It really helps me to know I can always take a PRN (as-needed) medication, stay on the phone with my daughter, or rely on my backup plan if I get too anxious. Are you suggesting that I give up these coping skills? Why would you even suggest this? If I did not have these to rely on, I would never do anything that makes me anxious.*

Answer—The goal is to eventually give up these kinds of "coping skills," which are actually safety behaviors. They are ways to avoid short-term discomfort, which paradoxically reinforces anticipatory anxiety in the long run. Asking you to give these up does not initially seem sensible—until you understand the processes that maintain anticipatory anxiety. Then it makes perfect sense. The partial and temporary relief you get from these workarounds actually reinforces the anxiety itself. And they rob you of the experience of discovering that you can indeed master what you are reluctant to face. Safety behaviors can be used as crutches: at the beginning of recovering, they may help you make the transition to self-reliance. But like any crutch, using them for too long holds you back and prevents you from learning what happens when you set out on your own.

Question—*What about breathing? I have always been taught to use breathing techniques to lower my anxiety. Why don't you talk about this in your book?*

Answer—Over the years, there have been a variety of recommendations about breathing. We are sure that many of you have been taught breathing techniques to reduce anxiety. So let's try to sort them out and see how they can be most helpful.

When you are feeling mild to moderate levels of anticipatory anxiety, calm breathing can slow down the nervous system and reduce physical arousal. There are numerous methods and apps available for practicing patterns of slow exhalation breathing that can be helpful. In fact, contrary to what you might have been advised, it is less important to breathe abdominally than to allow natural rhythmic breathing and full exhalations before inhaling once again. Pauses between breaths are helpful, but please don't try to breathe to a specific count. Deep sighing breaths that take in a lot of air are not recommended.

We are not against attending to the breath—both as a regular daily practice and during periods of increased anticipatory anxiety. We do, however, regularly see patients attempting to use breathing techniques in an utterly unhelpful way and want to caution readers about this. Many report that focusing on their breath makes them overly self-conscious of breathing and actually increases their anxiety by dysregulating their breathing more. When this happens, it can sometimes add to hyperventilation-induced (overbreathing) symptoms.

The intention of the breathwork is the key. If you are breathing in a relaxed or natural manner *while* you are experiencing anxiety or any other unwanted emotion, it can reduce a sense of urgency and remind you not to recoil from or avoid the experience you are having. It is grounding in the present moment sensory experience *while* allowing your mind and sensations and feelings to be what they are.

If, however, you are focusing on your breathing with the intention of changing, fixing, or getting away from your anxiety, then it becomes just another safety behavior or experiential avoidance method that interferes with learning. It has only a temporary effect and results in the negative reinforcement of your anxiety. Breathing is therefore not a helpful way to manage a full-fledged panic attack. Once again, any tool or technique used *in order* to lower anxiety, especially if used urgently, tends to backfire.

It may seem like a subtle distinction, but calming breathing can be part of the DANCE, or it can be in direct opposition to DANCE depending on your attitude and relationship to it. It can be a part of willingness and therapeutic surrender, or it can be utilized to undermine it.

Question—*It seems like you are telling me to make decisions impulsively and just live with the consequences. I am not willing to take the chance that I would be responsible for something bad that I could have prevented. I could never live with myself. If I stop worrying about consequences, what stops me from making mistakes?*

Answer—In real life, everyone makes mistakes. And everyone would like to make as few of them as possible with as few disastrous consequences as well. Moving forward in life requires the willingness to take reasonable risks and make commonsense decisions. None of us can predict the future, and we encourage reasonable fact-finding, research, and planning. There is nothing impulsive about that.

It sounds like you are overly focused on the possible negative consequences of a wrong decision. There are many uncertainties in life, and there is simply no way to ensure that bad things won't happen. After doing our research, we can only rely on making our best guess, guided by our own good judgment.

We all have our own definition of what constitutes sufficient research, but when you find yourself repeatedly going over the same or similar information, stretching deadlines to get in just one more bit of information, or paralyzed, unable to make a choice, this is no longer helpful. It is indecisiveness. You also have to consider the risks and costs of inaction—refusing or delaying a choice, missing a deadline, or the possibility of something going terribly wrong because you *didn't make a timely* decision.

Remember that making thoughtful, researched, and well-planned choices is the opposite of being impulsive. But that still doesn't eliminate the possibility of making a mistake, even a bad one. You are imagining that you could never survive being responsible for a bad outcome, and this is a story you are telling yourself, and you are then buying into that narrative. You can likely find in your past some regrets, mistakes, and unwelcome experiences that you might have prevented had you known what you know now, but you have dealt with these events and moved on.

Question—*I am a planner. I always know what I will do or say in the event of things going wrong. I feel better when I have reviewed in my mind as many scenarios as I can imagine before I set out to have a difficult conversation or do something anxiety producing. This gives me confidence. What is wrong with this? I believe it helps me.*

Answer—Let's not confuse planning and rehearsing with obsessing about possible bad outcomes and compulsively searching for a way to avoid them. If you are struggling with high anticipatory anxiety, somewhere along the way, your reasonable preparation has become hijacked by your vivid imagination. Although this overthinking may make you feel safer to undertake a particular challenging activity, in the long run, it undermines confidence in your ability to think on your feet, flexibly adjust to circumstances, or manage whatever might happen that you have not thought about. The more you overplan, the more you convince yourself that you need to.

Scenario-imagining or script-planning is an attempt to avoid being aware that you cannot know for sure what will happen. It reinforces the illusion that we can know the future. It gives a false sense of certainty. We are not suggesting that all preparation is counterproductive. Having a plan A and even a plan B can be useful. But attempting to cover all possibilities is impossible and exhausting. Then not having planned *enough* can, by itself, become the focus of your worries and stimulate more doubts. Trying to cover all potential scenarios leaves you with a set of inflexible *imagined solutions* instead of a willingness to innovate when spontaneous issues pop up.

Question—*I exercise daily, do mindfulness meditation, and drink chamomile tea nightly, and yet I am still sensitized. I have anticipatory anxiety whenever I am facing anything new or different. What else can I do to manage my stress level? Do you believe in supplements? How about acupuncture or yoga? Maybe I should change my job?*

Answer—Anticipatory anxiety is certainly stress-sensitive, which means that conflict, illness, sleep deprivation, and other forms of psychological and physiological stress will increase sensitization and stickiness of the mind. However, stress is not the cause of anticipatory anxiety, and reducing stress will not make it disappear. The factors that maintain anticipatory anxiety have to be addressed in order to be on the path to recovery. Your relationship to the experience of anxiety, your metacognitive beliefs, the presence of paradoxical effort, your willingness to experience uncertainty, and abandoning avoidance as a strategy for managing discomfort— all these factors are part of the program. Healthy habits are always welcome, but an all-out effort bent on avoiding stress is taking you in the wrong direction.

Question—*I am confused about refocusing attention. Isn't that distraction, and isn't distraction avoidance? And should you refocus on your present senses or on something calming, like imagining I am on the beach? The same with labeling something. If I tell myself that my worries are just a story I am making up, then isn't this reassurance, which I am not supposed to do? And what is the difference between floating and ignoring?*

Answer—These are great questions: they show you are reading and thinking carefully, and these questions are probably the most common requests for clarifications we get. There are lots of self-help books available, and some of them offer excellent suggestions for coping with anxiety. But sometimes their methods seem to clash, so let's try to sort out what is most helpful. Some common suggestions for managing anxiety are misguided. For example, trying to relax or thinking positive thoughts will not lead to lasting results. Other techniques have very limited value because they focus on controlling anxiety, either by distracting or avoiding, without addressing the enduring attitudinal factors. If you only look at *technique* instead of *process*, gains may be very temporary.

Often, the essential issue is not *what* you do, but rather your *intention* for doing it. If you refocus your attention in order to lower your anticipatory anxiety, then that is an attempt at distraction—you are trying to avoid the anxiety—which almost always backfires. However, if, for example, you become anxious while waiting to board a ski lift, and you refocus your attention on your present experiential reality while continuing to allow the feelings of anxiety, then that is much more therapeutic in the long run.

As you focus on your present experiences, your catastrophic anticipatory imaginings do not stop. That is not your goal. Instead, you are widening your perspective by including your present sensory realities so the anxious story becomes just one element—a single channel in the broadband of your awareness.

Labeling is quite similar. Once again, the purpose of labeling is not to lower your anxiety level. If you use it the way you describe in your question ("It's just a story…so I shouldn't worry about it"), you are reassuring yourself. And we know that repeated reassurance actually energizes anticipatory anxiety in the long run. Labeling therefore becomes a False Comfort compulsive ritual if you are applying it this way. Then, Worried Voice starts complaining that what you are worrying about could come true and needs attention. And you are back in the loop.

The primary purpose of labeling is to help you create and maintain the metacognitive perspective that *disentangles you from the content* of your thoughts. It allows you to step back and notice that "this is a thought." That is all. It has nothing to do with whether the thought is true or what the thought is about. It reminds you that you are reacting to a product of your own mind. This is not an anxiety management technique, but a necessary shift in perspective.

Finally, let's look at the distinction between floating and ignoring. Here the issue is differentiating between allowing and trying to push away. Floating (Weekes 1969) is a metaphor to describe the attitude of surrender. It comes from the fact that the best thing to do when feeling anxious is also one of the hardest things: do nothing. Yes, anticipatory anxiety goes down rather quickly if you just leave it alone and let your body calm down on its own. Floating is an entirely passive experience, like a cork bobbing on the water.

Ignoring, on the other hand, requires effort and energy. It is an action of pushing away something you already have perceived. This triggers paradoxical effort and ultimately acts to add to your anticipatory anxiety. Remember that effort works backward when dealing with anxiety: the more effort you put into struggling with anxiety, the stronger and stickier it becomes.

Question—*After I make any sort of decision, I am immediately haunted by the worry that I may have made a mistake. These doubts plague me for big things and little things, stuff I did yesterday and things from years ago that I can barely remember. How can I reassure myself that it will be okay?*

Answer—The fear that you might have made the wrong decision is potent fuel for chronic indecisiveness. Some people with chronic indecisiveness stay frozen at a choice point, unable to proceed at all. You seem to be able to make a choice, but then experience a particular kind of anticipatory anxiety: the fear *of regret*. Your imagination takes over, and you imagine all the things that could go wrong having made that decision, as well as all the options that you have eliminated by making that particular choice.

You ask how you can reassure yourself that all will be okay. The answer is that looking for reassurance is like starting a journey in the wrong direction. Instead of trying to reassure away your doubts, do the opposite: expect them, allow them, and welcome them. Understand that after you make each decision, you will indeed be seized with doubts. In an earlier chapter, we suggest counting your doubts and celebrating your creativity. Practice becoming more comfortable with the experience of uncertainty. Surrender to the impossibility of knowing the future for sure. Apply the steps of DANCE. Let your doubts and worries recede naturally to the background as you go on with your life.

CHAPTER 10

What Recovery Looks Like

You now understand much about anticipatory anxiety: what it is, how it happens, and how to shift your relationship with it so it no longer rules your life and determines your choices. It should therefore come as no surprise that recovery does not mean "no anticipatory anxiety anymore." Decades ago, Claire Weekes (1969) described recovery as "when symptoms no longer matter." This is a truly transformative statement: anxious arousal and worried thoughts do not have to be eliminated in order to become utterly irrelevant to your life.

Anticipatory anxiety or indecisiveness can show up any time, particularly when sensitized or under pressure. But you don't have to accept it as a reason for suffering, an occasion for self-reproach, or as guidance about future actions. Productively coping with anticipatory anxiety gives you the opportunity to choose your own path, unencumbered by anxious limitations. You will have flights of imagination about what might happen and what could have happened that will become momentarily upsetting, annoying, irrelevant, absurd, and even comical. You will be able to give a nod to your creativity and step back into ordinary reality.

In a similar way, as you become more flexible, less perfectionistic, and more willing to notice uncertainty and doubts, decisions will become simpler. The potential for regret will be acknowledged but not paralyzing. Endless research, reassurance-seeking, and hesitations will fade. You will be able to move forward with your best guesses where you are stuck.

Recovery means being disentangled from the content of your anxious imaginings and unfazed by the appearance of anxious thoughts, sensations, and feelings. It means acknowledging past discomforts without letting them stop you. It does not mean never making up anxious stories automatically or hesitating to make a choice. It certainly doesn't mean being immune to worries.

Finally, recovery does not mean being impulsive or becoming an unreasonable risk-taker. It just means recognizing what is happening when you have anticipatory anxiety, being kind to yourself, and not letting the pull of avoidance limit your life.

DANCE is not a sequence of actions designed to be activated in case anticipatory anxiety arises. It is not a technique in a bag of tools. It is a profound shift in your response to anxious thoughts, feelings, and sensations, which may arise from memories, imagination, mood, or automatic conditioned habits of the mind. With practice, this shift becomes a natural process. It is a way of living your life as it unfolds.

When Anticipatory Anxiety Fades, Excitement Reemerges

Sigmund Freud, the father of psychoanalysis, made the astute observation about people who suffered from severe anxiety: he noted that prior to developing anxiety about them, these same objects and experiences elicited pleasure and excitement. He noted the relationship between excitement and anxiety (Freud 1964).

Years ago, a group of very anxious patients in Baltimore went with their therapist to ride elevators and face their fears. There was nothing but dread as the group fell silent, waiting in the hotel lobby for the high-speed glass-walled elevator to arrive. As they stepped on, clutching each other's hands for support, they were greeted by a man who had boarded from the parking area below. Just as the elevator took off, this man turned to the group with a beaming smile and said, "Don't you just love the rush?"

Yes, anticipation can sometimes become pleasurable, not just tolerable. This "rush" is called excitement, and it can be what you feel as you wait for awards to be announced, as you log on to the dating website, or when someone suggests going on a vacation. It is physiological arousal for sure, but it is not distressing. It is what people pay for when they ride roller coasters and when they go to a sports event where they really care about who wins. It is the stimulated nervous system of a person walking down the aisle to get married or waiting at the corner where they will meet their date for the first time.

HELPFUL FACT—Anticipation can become "looking forward to," excitement, or just fun.

False "Warnings" from the Past Will Happen During Recovery

Anticipatory anxiety is frequently the "last to go" during the process of recovery from most anxiety disorders and obsessive-compulsive disorders. Long after you are no longer having panic attacks and you have been facing your fears for months, and long after you no longer need to perform compulsive rituals and have stopped turning to False Comfort for help, there is often a lingering anticipatory anxiety. Zelda Milstein (1983), a pioneering paraprofessional therapist who recovered from ten years of being housebound with agoraphobia using the methods of Claire Weekes, told her patients that she frequently had a predictable blip of anxiety right when she crossed the threshold of her front door. She called it "the hump" and talked about it as a false warning leftover. It is a conditioned response with a long half-life and is best celebrated as the body's memory and evidence of what you have overcome.

It is important not to be discouraged when this or any other anxiety symptom shows up. It is just part of the process. It is also important not to get lost in the "why" when this happens. Automatic arousal and instant anxious stories can simply be allowed to remain present in the background of your experience. When you are disentangled from what they might mean, you do not struggle against them, you simply accept them as evidence of how far you have come, that you remain on the path to recovery, and that you are rewiring your brain's circuitry.

HELPFUL FACT—When anxiety comes back, don't get caught up in "Why?" Simply, gently, return to the DANCE.

To reiterate: recovering is not about *not* experiencing anticipatory anxiety; it is about changing your relationship with it. Take victory laps for not avoiding when you want to, for embracing discomfort when you could have taken an easier route, for making a choice even while feeling uncertain. The most enduring progress happens when the circumstances are difficult and your catastrophic predictions are challenged. This means that episodes of setbacks or old patterns reemerging are the best opportunities to continue to consolidate what you are learning.

Building Confidence

Anxiety specialist Jonathan Dalton (2021) shared this story in his workshops:

> *Imagine an eagle sitting high up on a branch of a tree. He notices a crack in the branch. Why is he not scared? Is it because he is reassuring himself that the crack is small or that his weight won't affect it? Or is he telling himself that the chances are very small that it will break today? No. He is not scared because he knows he can fly.*

Understanding anticipatory anxiety is certainly a prerequisite for recovery. But what grows your confidence and motivates you to keep moving ahead is watching yourself as you stop avoiding anxious experiences and come through discomfort intact. Remember that action precedes motivation, confidence, and comfort. There are no guarantees that bad things can't happen or that you won't get rejected or stumble or regret a decision, but like the eagle, when you know you can fly, you are ready to handle whatever arises.

As we have described, building confidence comes from observing yourself bravely moving onward. This means proceeding with action *before* "being sure" you will succeed. Each time you manage to avoid avoidance, you are constructing your new relationship with yourself—one in which you stay grounded in the present moment, you are kind to yourself about being anxious, and you demonstrate that you can do it no matter how you feel. Anticipatory anxiety and chronic indecisiveness can no longer bully you. They may show up, but you give them no power.

Your Personal Recovery Letter

When you have accomplished something big that you had antici-pated with elaborate dread, here is something very important for you to do. It is so easy to be hijacked by your imagination, and our minds are primed to remember the distress of anticipation and forget successes. So we recommend that you write a personal letter to your future self (or, if you prefer, make a video recording or a journal blog) in which you speak to yourself compassionately about what you did, what you decided, or what challenge you met even while being aware of having anticipatory anxiety. Be clear that this was not easy but that the shift to DANCE was worth it.

Tell your future self how you were able to proceed. Write a letter to your future self, who will be reading this letter perhaps while being caught up in catastrophizing and ruminating and debating acts of avoidance, to remind yourself not to believe what you are thinking. Tell your future self not to buy into the stories you are creating about possibilities instead of probabilities and not to assume that the anxiety you feel is a warning or a prediction. Even more importantly, tell your future self that you have shown how you can indeed handle anxiety without letting it stop you, even though you might believe that you cannot stand it, and what freedom and flexibility feel like on the other side. Then put this letter to your future self in a place where you come across it regularly so you will remember it at some point in the future when you will benefit from reading it.

No One Is Entirely Free of Anticipatory Anxiety

We have emphasized that while you are working on your anticipatory anxiety, avoidance—both experiential and behavioral—sets you back and reinforces anxiety. But after recovery, there are plenty of times when you might choose to avoid, even though you are making a less anxious choice.

For example, if, during the process of recovery, you have been deliber-ately choosing the long line in the supermarket in order to practice waiting in line with anticipatory anxiety about the interaction with the cashier, eventually this will no longer be necessary. Most people choose the short line; if they have no option but the long line, they know they can manage it and, perhaps with a short blip of anticipatory anxiety, step confidently into the "trap" of the line.

It is tempting to be perfectionistic about recovery, but that can get in your way and reduce enjoyment of your gains. Here is a dialogue among our voices who are well into recovery and living a full life.

Worried Voice: I thought I was over anticipatory anxiety. I really don't avoid anything I want to do anymore. Now, I am suddenly hesitating to commit to that vacation we have been planning because of the hurricane season. What if the weather ruins everything? I have to commit, right? What if I give in to my worries? Will I just slide backward about everything? What is wrong with me?

False Comfort: Hurricanes are spotted days ahead of time. And the hotel is new and strong. We should just grit our teeth and send the money. Give in to avoidance once and it will take over. This is definitely the right thing to do. We have to face our fears, right? No matter how we feel, right? We'll be okay if we just commit.

Worried Voice: Okay, but are we allowed to get those refundable tickets during hurricane season? Or is that a sign of relapse?

Wise Mind: Let me step in here. Recovery is flexibility, not rigid rules. Old habits of the mind will pop up from time to time. You were well conditioned to pay too much attention to pop-up worries. You regularly got derailed by your catastrophic thinking. Now you don't do that very often. But that does not mean that no doubts can ever be considered. You do not have to be perfect.

You began worrying about your worries as soon as you noticed some doubts. Worried Voice focused on "What is wrong with me?" and "What if this is relapse?" False Comfort fell back on the old habit of empty reassurance.

Everyone occasionally gets some anticipatory anxiety and has some doubts. This is part of life. You can note it, address it, accept it with self-compassion, decide what to do, and then move on.

Conclusion

You now recognize some essential facts about your anticipatory anxiety.

- You are not required to take the stories of your imagination, memories, or worries as serious warnings or predictions. You do not have to believe what you are thinking.

- You can observe without judgment. You can get past self-criticism. You can proceed toward doing what matters, even while feeling the physiology of arousal and the clanging of false alarms.

- You are making decisions and choices with reasonable ease, even as you are aware of doubts, imperfections, and the possibility that you might experience regret. You are not constantly stuck in ambivalence, research, or procrastination.

- You are building confidence by doing things that challenge you, not by waiting for confidence before you do them. You can genuinely celebrate your flexibility and freedom.

Worried Voice: I don't feel anxious every day! How amazing.

False Comfort: And it is okay not to worry.

Wise Mind: Yes indeed.

Postscript

Once you no longer need to avoid and know how to DANCE with flexibility and confidence, you can apply the wisdom attributed to E. L. Doctorow to your own anticipatory anxieties and chronic indecisiveness. As Anne

Lamott (1994) reports it in her book *Bird by Bird,* Doctorow once said, "Writing a novel is like driving a car at night. You can see only as far as your headlights, but you can make the whole trip that way" (18).

"You don't have to see where you're going," Lamott adds, "you don't have to see your destination or everything you will pass along the way. You just have to see two or three feet ahead of you. This is right up there with the best advice on writing, or life, I have ever heard" (18).

Acknowledgments

Every time we are working on a book, I declare definitively that this is the last book, and then just as we are finishing it, Marty has yet another idea for the next book and starts campaigning. Thank you. For years of friendship and collaborative thinking on Google Docs where we edit, delete, and clarify each other's words even as we are writing them. I also want to tell everyone that he is the one who manages all the technological demands of doing this work as I studiously avoid learning how to do them.

I particularly want to thank Michael Heady and Sarah Crawley for shouldering much of my share of the work involved in keeping our Anxiety and Stress Disorders Institute going. And I value the education I so often receive in conversation with our training director Carl Robbins. I also want to acknowledge the enthusiasm and professionalism we have received at all levels from New Harbinger Publications.

This manuscript was written during the pandemic while we all faced daily uncertainties and anxious imaginings. I want to thank my Zoom communities—professional, friends, and family—for staying connected and giving enough of the illusion of "normal" to be able to manage. I am grateful for having had the privilege to be in a pod with one daughter's family while my other daughters have been in two other countries with closed borders. I am incredibly grateful to the people who delivered my groceries; pursued scientific, social justice, and public health objectives; and took care of us all.

—Sally Winston, June 2021

This book is the third of a trilogy. When we began writing our book on intrusive thoughts, we weren't yet clear that the anxious experience has three separate components, each of which deserve a self-help volume. It fell upon me to convince Sally to complete the trilogy because there is no way I could have done it on my own. I am so pleased by our long-term friendship, our affection, and even our style of arguing. If I am the techno-nerd, then Sally is the more creative, thoughtful, and knowledgeable one. We are an excellent team—each of us providing what the other does not. I am thrilled that our writings have helped so many, and our two previous books have been translated into a total of eleven languages over the past year.

And what a year this has been! Throughout the pandemic and political turmoil, I have been blessed with great friends and family. I thank Ruta for her support, her attention, and her love, and Eva for joining the family. My cycling pod has gotten me through the worst of the isolation, and I thank Kathy, Yvonne, Peter, Michele, and John for keeping me active and engaged. A special thanks to my patients who—especially during this time—have taught me far more than any of my book learning. And to Carl for cogent clarification on some important issues. Thank you also, New Harbinger Publications, for your timely assistance in guiding this book to completion: Jess, Vicraj, and Gretel.

—Martin Seif, June 2021

References

Amir, N., M. Freshman, B. Ramsey, E. Neary, and B. Brigidi. 2001. "Thought-Action Fusion in Individuals with OCD Symptoms." *Behaviour Research and Therapy* 39, no. 7: 765–776.

Arco, A. D., and F. Mora. 2009. "Neurotransmitters and Prefrontal Cortex–Limbic System Interactions: Implications for Plasticity and Psychiatric Disorders." *Journal of Neural Transmissions* 116: 941–952.

Carbonell, D. A. 2016. *The Worry Trick: How Your Brain Tricks You into Expecting the Worst and What You Can Do About It*. Oakland, CA: New Harbinger Publications.

Chesterton, G. K. 1956. *What's Wrong with This World*. New York: Sheed and Ward.

Craske, M. G., M. Treanor, C. C. Conway, T. Zbozinek, and B. Vervliet. 2014. "Maximizing Exposure Therapy: An Inhibitory Learning Approach." *Behaviour Research and Therapy* 58: 10–23.

Dalton, J. 2021. "The Use of Metaphor in Translating Complicated Clinical Concepts into Relatable Language." ADAA. March 19, 2021 (virtual workshop).

Davis, W. E., S. Abney, S. Perekslis, S-L. Eshun, and R. Dunn. 2018. "Multidimensional Perfectionism and Perceptions of Potential Relationship Partners." *Personality and Individual Differences* 127: 31–38.

Eaton, W. W., D. A Regier, B. Z. Locke, and C. A. Taube. 1981. "The Epidemiologic Catchment Area Program of the National Institute of Mental Health." *Public Health Reports* 96, no. 4: 319–325.

Freeston, M. H., M. J. Dugas, and R. Ladouceur. 1996. "Thoughts, Images, Worry, and Anxiety." *Cognitive Therapy and Research* 20, no. 3: 265–273.

Freud, S. 1964. *The Standard Edition of the Complete Psychological Works of Sigmund Freud,* edited by J. Strachey. New York: Macmillan.

Fried, R., and J. Grimaldi. 1993. "Respiration, Hyperventilation, and Mental Disorders." In *The Psychology and Physiology of Breathing.* *The Springer Series in Behavioral Psychophysiology and Medicine.* Boston, MA: Springer.

Garrido, M. I., G. R. Barnes, M. Sahani, and R. J. Dolan. 2012. "Functional Evidence for a Dual Route to Amygdala." *Current Biology* 22, no. 2: 129–134.

Grayson, J. 2014. *Freedom from Obsessive-Compulsive Disorder: A Personalized Recovery Program for Living with Uncertainty.* New York: Berkley Books.

Greenberg, M. J. 2021. "Why Rumination Is a Continuous Loop." https://drmichaeljgreenberg.com/why-rumination-is-a-continuous-loop/.

Grupe, D. W., and J. B. Nitschke. 2013. "Uncertainty and Anticipation in Anxiety: An Integrated Neurobiological and Psychological Perspective." *Nature Reviews Neuroscience* 14, no. 7: 488–501.

Harris, R. 2017. "Nuts and Bolts of Creative Hopelessness." https://www.actmindfully.com.au/upimages/Nuts_and_Bolts_of_Creative_Hopelessness_-_May_2017_version.pdf.

Harris, R. 2019. *ACT Made Simple: An Easy-to-Read Primer on Acceptance and Commitment Therapy.* Oakland, CA: New Harbinger Publications.

Helbig-Lang, S., T. Lang, F. Petermann, and J. Hoyer. 2012. "Anticipatory Anxiety as a Function of Panic Attacks and Panic-Related Self-Efficacy: An Ambulatory Assessment Study in Panic Disorder." *Behavioural and Cognitive Psychotherapy* 40, no. 5: 590–604.

Hewitt, P., C. Chen, M. Smith, L. Zhang, M. Habke, G. Flett, and S. Mikail. 2019. "Patient Perfectionism and Clinician Impression Formation During an Initial Interview." *Psychology and Psychotherapy Theory Research and Practice* 94, no. 1: 45–62.

Hoare, J. 2019. "Face, Accept, Float, Let Time Pass: Claire Weekes' Anxiety Cure Holds True Decades On." *Sidney Morning Tribune*. September 21, 2019. https://www.smh.com.au/lifestyle/health-and -wellness/face-accept-float-let-time-pass-claire-weekes-anxiety-cure -holds-true-decades-on-20190917-p52s2w.html.

Kensinger, E. A. 2009. "Remembering the Details: Effects of Emotion." *Emotion Review* 1, no. 2: 99–113.

Kerr, E. 2020. "Colleges with the Highest Application Fees." US News Education, November 24. https://www.usnews.com/education/best -colleges/the-short-list-college/articles/colleges-with-the-highest -application-fees.

Koffka, K. 1935. *Principles of Gestalt Psychology*. New York: Harcourt, Brace, and Company.

Lamott, A. 1994. *Bird by Bird: Some Instructions on Writing and Life*. New York: Anchor Books.

Milstein, Z. Personal communication. September 1983.

O'Connor, K., F. Aardema, and M-C. Pélissier. 2005. *Beyond Reasonable Doubt: Reasoning Processes in Obsessive-Compulsive Disorder and Related Disorders*. Hoboken, NJ: John Wiley & Sons.

Pittman, C. M., and E. M. Karle. 2015. *Rewire Your Anxious Brain: How to Use the Neuroscience of Fear to End Anxiety, Panic, and Worry*. Oakland, CA: New Harbinger Publications.

Rajmohan, V., and E. Mohandas. 2007. "The Limbic System." *Indian Journal of Psychiatry* 49, no. 2: 132–139. https://doi.org/10 .4103/0019-5545.33264.

Robbins, C. Personal communication. March 2016.

Salkovskis, P. M. 1985. "Obsessional-Compulsive Problems: A Cognitive-Behavioural Analysis." *Behaviour Research and Therapy* 23, no. 5: 571–583.

Scott, E. 2020. "What Is the Law of Attraction?" Very Well Mind. https:// www.verywellmind.com/understanding-and-using-the-law -of-attraction-3144808.

Seif, M. N., and S. Winston. 2014. *What Every Therapist Needs to Know About Anxiety Disorders: Key Concepts, Insights, and Interventions.* New York: Routledge.

Seif, M. N., and S. Winston. 2019. *Needing to Know for Sure: A CBT-Based Guide to Overcoming Compulsive Checking and Reassurance Seeking.* Oakland, CA: New Harbinger Publications.

Sewart, A. R., and M. G. Craske. 2020. "Inhibitory Learning." In *Clinical Handbook of Fear and Anxiety: Maintenance Processes and Treatment Mechanisms,* edited by J. S. Abramowitz and S. M. Blakey. Washington, DC: American Psychological Association.

Singh, P., S. S. Yoon, and B. Kuo. 2016. "Nausea: A Review of Pathophysiology and Therapeutics." *Therapeutic Advances in Gastroenterology* 9, no. 1: 98–112.

Straube, T., S. Schmidt, T. Weiss, H. J. Mentzel, and W. H. Miltner. 2009. "Dynamic Activation of the Anterior Cingulate Cortex During Anticipatory Anxiety." *Neuroimage* 44, no. 3: 975–981.

Tavel, M. E. 2017. "Hyperventilation Syndrome: A Diagnosis Usually Unrecognized." *Journal of Internal Medicine and Primary Healthcare* 2, no. 1: 1–4.

Wang, Y., A. Luppi, J. Fawcett, and M. C. Anderson. 2019. "Reconsidering Unconscious Persistence: Suppressing Unwanted Memories Reduces Their Indirect Expression in Later Thoughts." *Cognition* 187: 78–94.

Weekes, C. 1969. *Hope and Help for Your Nerves.* New York: Hawthorne Books.

Winston, S., and M. Seif. 2017. *Overcoming Unwanted Intrusive Thoughts: A CBT-Based Guide to Getting Over Frightening, Obsessive, or Disturbing Thoughts.* Oakland, CA: New Harbinger Publications.

Wu, M., D. S. Mennin, M. Ly, H. T. Karim, L. Banihashemi, D. L. Tudorascu, H. J. Aizenstein, and C. Andreescu. 2019. "When Worry May Be Good for You: Worry Severity and Limbic-Prefrontal Functional Connectivity in Late-Life Generalized Anxiety Disorder." *Journal of Affective Disorders* 257: 650–657.

Sally M. Winston, PsyD, is founder and executive director of the Anxiety and Stress Disorders Institute in Baltimore, MD. She is a founding clinical fellow of the Anxiety and Depression Association of America (ADAA), winner of the inaugural ADAA Jerilyn Ross Award, and was previously awarded the Association for Behavioral and Cognitive Therapies (ABCT) book award. She has over forty years of clinical practice and training specializing in anxiety disorders and obsessive-compulsive disorder (OCD). She is coauthor, with Martin Seif, of *What Every Therapist Needs to Know About Anxiety Disorders*, *Overcoming Unwanted Intrusive Thoughts*, and *Needing to Know for Sure*.

Martin N. Seif, PhD, is cofounder of the ADAA, and was a member of its board of directors for fourteen years. Seif was associate director of The Anxiety and Phobia Treatment Center at White Plains Hospital, a faculty member of New York-Presbyterian Hospital, and is board certified in cognitive behavioral therapy (CBT) from the American Board of Professional Psychology. He was previously awarded the ABCT book award, and maintains a private practice in Greenwich, CT. He is coauthor, with Sally Winston, of *What Every Therapist Needs to Know About Anxiety Disorders*, *Overcoming Unwanted Intrusive Thoughts*, and *Needing to Know for Sure*.

Real change *is* possible

For more than forty-five years, New Harbinger has published proven-effective self-help books and pioneering workbooks to help readers of all ages and backgrounds improve mental health and well-being, and achieve lasting personal growth. In addition, our spirituality books offer profound guidance for deepening awareness and cultivating healing, self-discovery, and fulfillment.

Founded by psychologist Matthew McKay and Patrick Fanning, New Harbinger is proud to be an independent, employee-owned company. Our books reflect our core values of integrity, innovation, commitment, sustainability, compassion, and trust. Written by leaders in the field and recommended by therapists worldwide, New Harbinger books are practical, accessible, and provide real tools for real change.

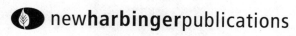 **newharbinger**publications

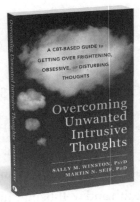
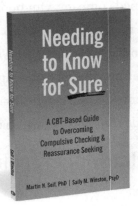
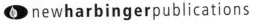